INTERNATIONAL PERSPECTIVES IN PHY

Pain

SERIES EDITORS

Ida Bromley MBE MCSP

Ida Bromley is District Superintendent Physiotherapist at The Royal Free Hospital, London. A Superintendent Physiotherapist for the past 20 years in hospitals in England, she has lectured and run workshops in various parts of the U.K., U.S.A. and South Africa, and written articles for many journals on subjects ranging from 'Rehabilitation of the Severely Disabled' to 'Problem Orientated Medical Recording'. She is also author of a well-known textbook, *Tetraplegia and Paraplegia*. From 1978–82, she was Chairman of the Council of the Chartered Society of Physiotherapy and is currently President of the Organisation of District Physiotherapists and Vice-President of the Society for Research in Rehabilitation.

Nancy Theilgaard Watts RPT PhD

Nancy Watts is Professor and Director of the Physical Therapy Graduate Program in the MGH Institute of Health Professions at Massachusetts General Hospital in Boston. A physical therapy teacher for over 30 years, since 1965 most of her work has been in establishing advanced study programs for experienced therapists. Her major academic interests and publications concern methods of clinical teaching, economics of health care, and analysis of the process of judgment used by clinicians. Her clinical research has varied widely, ranging from studies of the effects of cold on spasticity to cost-effectiveness comparisons of different methods of treatment for common orthopaedic disorders. Dr Watts has served on a number of national and international commissions, and frequently teaches and consults in Britain, Scandinavia, and Latin America. She has also helped to prepare physical therapy teachers for schools in over 20 different countries.

INTERNATIONAL PERSPECTIVES IN PHYSICAL THERAPY 1

Pain

EDITED BY

Theresa Hoskins Michel MS RPT

Assistant Professor,
Program in Physical Therapy,
Institute of Health Professions,
Massachusetts General Hospital;
Clinical Specialist in Cardiopulmonary Physical Therapy,
Massachusetts General Hospital, Massachusetts, USA

FOREWORD BY

Beverly Bishop PhD
Professor of Physiology,
State University of New York, Buffalo, NY, USA

CHURCHILL LIVINGSTONE
EDINBURGH LONDON MELBOURNE AND NEW YORK 1985

CHURCHILL LIVINGSTONE
Medical Division of Longman Group Limited

Distributed in the United States of America by
Churchill Livingstone Inc., 1560 Broadway, New York,
N.Y. 10036, and by associated companies, branches
and representatives throughout the world.

First published 1985

ISBN 0 443 02922 9

ISSN 0267-0380

British Library Cataloguing in Publication Data
Pain. — (International perspectives in
  physical therapy; 1)
  1. Pain
  I. Michel, Theresa Hoskins   II. Series
  616'.0472   RB127

Library of Congress Cataloging in Publication Data
Main entry under title:
Pain.
  (International perspectives in physical therapy;
v. 1)
  Bibliography: p.
  Includes index.
  1. Pain — Treatment. 2. Pain — Physiological aspects.
3. Physical therapy. I. Michel, Theresa Hoskins.
II. Series. [DNLM: 1. Pain — therapy. W1 IN827JM v.1/
WL 704 P1441]
RB127.P3315   1985   616'.0472   84–23895

Produced by Longman Singapore Publishers (Pte) Limited
Printed in Singapore

About the Series

The purpose of this series of books is to provide an international exchange of ideas and to explore different approaches in professional therapy practice.

The books will be written primarily for experienced clinicians. They are not intended as basic texts nor as reports on the most recent research, though elements of these aspects may be included.

Articles written by experts from a number of different countries will form the core of each volume. These will be supported by a commentary on the current 'state of the art' in the particular area of practice and an annotated bibliography of key references.

Each volume will cover a topic which we believe to be of universal interest. Some will be concerned with a troublesome symptom, as in this volume; others will be related to problems within a broad diagnostic category, for example sports injuries. Aspects of the organisation of practice and issues of professional concern will be the subjects of future books in the series.

In this volume we have adopted the convention of using 'he' for patient and 'she' for physiotherapist.

We hope that readers will let us have their reactions to the content and format of these publications. Suggestions of other topics considered to be of international interest, which might provide the foci of future volumes would also be welcomed.

I.B
N.T.W

My special thanks go to my husband, Tony, and our two children, Joel and Sarah, who allowed me the peace-of-mind to do this work.

Foreword

Pain is man's most worrisome sensation. It is worrisome not only to the individual experiencing it but also to the clinician attempting to treat it and to the neuroscientist trying to elucidate its physiological and psychological mechanisms.

For centuries the subject of pain was too fragmented and sketchy to be synthesized into any comprehensive view. This situation has completely reversed since 1969 when Reynolds reported that he could perform abdominal surgery on rats without anesthesia by electrically stimulating the periaqueductal gray (PAG) matter in the brain stem. This observation, which has since been repeatedly confirmed, led rapidly to other equally important discoveries. Soon after, naloxone, a specific opiate antagonist, was shown to reduce the analgesic effects of PAG stimulation. Then the endogenous endorphins were discovered, and this in turn led to the discovery of opiate receptors and opioid peptide-containing neurons within those brain areas where electrical stimulation or microinjection of opiates would produce analgesia. These discoveries spawned new pharmaceutical agents designed to imitate the analgesic actions of the endogenous endorphins but lacking their addictive properties.

Equally important milestones contributing to an understanding of the basic properties of the nociceptive systems were the direct result of the Gate Control Theory put forth by Melzack and Wall in 1965 and reports about the miracles of acupuncture brought back by those who had visited China. From these provocative notions investigators evolved very fruitful hypotheses which were put to experimental test. Out of these endeavors came our current concepts about endorphin and non-endorphin pain-inhibiting systems of the nervous system. These discoveries were directly responsible for the introduction of a new treatment procedure into the physical therapist's regime, namely transcutaneous electrical nerve stimulation (TENS), and for the development of an industry to manufacture the stimulators.

New information about pain continues to evolve at such an accelerated rate that only specialists can keep pace. Many factors account for this rapid expansion of knowledge. Investigators representing a myriad of disciplines are combining their skills in unorthodox ways. Innovative methods are being developed for identifying neurons in the central nervous system which are involved in pain and for studying their intrinsic properties. Putative neurotransmitters with analgesic actions continue to be discovered. New ways of activating the descending pain-inhibiting systems are being sought. The research efforts expended to acquire this knowledge will reach full fruition when the new knowledge can be applied to prevent, reduce or abolish pain.

Despite this knowledge explosion about the neurophysiology, neurobiochemistry, neuropharmacology and neuroanatomy of pain, we are still many years away from knowing how best to utilize the new knowledge in the clinical setting. One important means for accelerating the dissemination of any new knowledge is via communication. Volume 1 on Pain in the series, *International Perspectives in Physical Therapy*, promises to provide an ideal mechanism for sharing new and established knowledge among physical therapists and other clinicians around the world.

I am flattered to have been asked to write this Foreword for Volume 1. It provides me with the opportunity to compliment the physical therapists on their objectives of keeping abreast of major topics intellectually as well as technically. This new international series should facilitate the exchange of ideas and assemble the most current information in the selected areas. My best wishes to them in this worthwhile endeavor.

Buffalo, N.Y., 1985   Beverly Bishop

Contributors

Darian Duffin MCSP, SRP, Lic Ac
Formerly Senior Physiotherapist, Physiotherapy Department, Royal Free Hospital, London, UK

Ruth-Randi Ellingsen Dip TP, Cert Spec Study
Senior Lecturer in Physical Therapy, Fysioterapihøgskolen, Oslo, Norway

Theresa Hoskins Michel MS, RPT
Assistant Professor, Program in Physical Therapy, Institute of Health Professions, Massachusetts General Hospital; Clinical Specialist in Cardiopulmonary Physical Therapy, Massachusetts General Hospital, Boston, Massachusetts, USA

Jeffrey S. Mannheimer MA, RPT
President, Delaware Valley Physical Therapy Associates, Lawrenceville, New Jersey; Clinical Assistant Professor, College of Allied Health Professions, Program in Physical Therapy, Hannemann University, Philadelphia, Pennsylvania; Instructor, College of Arts and Sciences, School of Life and Health Sciences, Allied Health Professions, University of Delaware, Newark, Delaware, USA

Margaret H. Moon MSc, NZRP
Psychologist, Physiotherapist, Relaxation and Biofeedback Centre, Christchurch, New Zealand

Gunilla Myrnerts Dip TP
Physiotherapist, Occupational Health and Safety Department, Saab Scania, Linköping, Sweden

Stanley V. Paris PhD, MCSP, NZSP, PT
Visiting Lecturer, Massachusetts General Hospital, Institute of Health Professions, Boston, Massachusetts; President, Institute of Graduate Health Sciences, Atlanta, Georgia, USA

Carol A. Ezzo Schaefer MS, RPT
Associate Professor of Physical Therapy, School of Health Related Professions, University of Mississippi Medical Center, Jackson, Mississippi, USA

Marit Østby Sundsvold Dip TP
Teacher in Postgraduate Education in Psychiatric/Psychosomatic Physiotherapy, Research Physiotherapist, Psychiatric Department, Ulleval University Hospital, Oslo, Norway

Per Vaglum MD, Dr Med
Professor of Psychiatry, University of Oslo, Oslo, Norway

Peter Wells MCSP, Dip TP
Superintendent Physiotherapist, St Stephen's Hospital, London, UK

June M. Williams BSc (PT), MSc (Clinical Neurology)
Assistant Professor, School of Physical and Occupational Therapy, McGill
University, Montreal, Canada

Contents

Introduction and state of the art

PAIN: THE CLINICAL PROBLEM

The clinical problem of pain is an especially perplexing and complex one, and in terms of physical therapy solutions perhaps one of our least successful areas of concern. Why is it that pain is still one of the most challenging clinical areas of physical therapy? Yet pain is perhaps the original symptom bringing the patient to the medical expert for advice or treatment. The answer to this question is elusive and obviously complex. Part of the reason must be in the inadequate depth of understanding of what pain is or what mechanisms underly the full pain experience. There are multiple ways to define pain, and each person or profession chooses to work with the definition which most adequately describes the pain with which they can best deal. Each professional group becomes locked into their own vocabulary of pain, and the ability to cross-fertilize experience or understanding may be limited by the language and concepts of the group. Sternbach, a prominent neurologist in the field of pain, has stated that pain is an abstract term which refers to many different phenomena from which one makes a selection, depending on whether one is giving neurological, physiological, behavioral, subjective or psychiatric descriptions (Sternbach, 1974). The theories of pain reflect this same plurality of definition.

Another answer to our question may lie in the problem that medical professionals tend to interpret all pain according to the rather limited model of acute pain which has a clear sensory component. Many types of pain have no obvious sensory configuration, but are described qualitatively rather than quantitatively. This is likely to be due to the reactive component of the pain experience. Pain is far more complex than a simple stimulus-response reflex, which is more typical of an acute pain situation. Psychosocial responses contribute to the experience of pain, which make it difficult to assess pain, treat pain and study the effects of treatment upon pain (Degenaar, 1979).

To give examples of the plurality of descriptions of pain, pain may be and has been defined in terms of: (1) nerve impules, (2) emotional qualities, (3) sensations, feelings, suffering, meaning and (4) guilt and punishment. In my exploration of physical therapy approaches to treatment of pain, I have found the entire spectrum, represented to a large degree by papers presented in this volume on Pain. I believe that it is ultimately more useful to us and to our patients to draw on as many of these models as possible, rather than to limit ourselves to one vocabulary, one theory or one treatment approach.

DEFINITIONS: TYPES OF PAIN

Acute pain

Clinical pain generally means either a symptom of a disease condition, or a temporary aspect of treatment. In both cases, patient and therapist hold an expectation of alleviation. Pain is perceived as a warning that something is wrong with the structural or functional integrity of the body. This perception creates a reaction to the acute pain, rendering the experience much more than the sensation of pain alone. The reaction component of pain is highly individual, subjective and experiential. But in acute pain, most often the cause of the pain is identifiable and self-limiting or correctable. The reaction to this type of pain results in typical patterns of response that restore the person to his natural equilibrium, for example, reflex muscle spasm and automatic splinting at a fracture site, or the avoidance of foods which would increase the pain of a stomach ulcer.

Chronic pain

Often acute pain leads into chronic pain, but chronic pain can also begin insidiously. At some point, the pain exists without any known time limit. Chronic pain becomes a constant companion, even when intermittent. It is likely to become inextricably intertwined into the person's personality. Sometimes the source of this pain is known but no treatment is available, or chronic pain may be of unknown etiology. The threat that chronic pain imposes on the person generates reaction patterns which are unpredictable, individual, and often very complex.

Intractable pain

When chronic pain persists even when treatment is provided, or when it exists without demonstrable disease, intractable pain is present. Intractable pain presents the greatest challenge to all health care providers in every dimension of the human experience.

PAIN EVALUATION

For physical therapists, one of the major obstacles to successful treatment of pain has been in evaluating pain in systematic, repeatable, objective ways. We observe our patients as they move to find their general mobility level and their ranges of pain-free motion. We ask them specific questions to determine their subjective experience of pain. We continue to find it difficult at times to differentiate real pain from malingering, or different types of real pain. Physical therapists are not unique in these problems. There are now available, more than ever before, questionnaires, rating scales, and other formats for the evaluation of pain, many of which are presented in this volume on Pain. The validity and reliability of each form should be established, and in many cases has been tested, to provide for us the level of confidence that we need to use such a form in our own clinical setting and trust in the results it gives us. Then we can make effective use of the information for two major purposes: (1) to help us decide upon our treatment goals and program; and (2) to provide a baseline for later comparisons if change occurs in a patient's pain, namely, change from our treatment or other intervention, from spontaneous remission or from progression of some disease.

The evaluation of pain should take into account five levels of the total pain experience (Johnson, 1977). As clinicians, we first determine whether or not pain exists. As I indicated, this is not always easy or even possible. A very skilled 'intractable malingerer' may be far more clever at convincing people than we give him credit for! New ingenious tests for this basic level of pain evaluation could be very helpful.

Once pain is identified, the second level is to evaluate the descriptive characteristics of pain. These include location, duration, pattern, triggering phenomena, intensity, quality. Besides a simple interview with the patient, the use of aforementioned rating scales or questionnaires can be extremely valuable. Observations of the patient and physiologic measurements provide the third level of pain evaluation; to determine what physiologic and behavioral responses are occurring with pain. Then the evaluation of the individual's perception of his pain and the meaning that his pain holds for him is a fourth level. This level, too, holds many challenges, and may be best assessed by more than one person in a team of health care providers dealing with one patient.

The final level to evaluate is that of determining what adaptive mechanisms are being used to cope with pain. There are 5 typical mechanisms useful to most individuals when facing any disaster: (1) denial (2) group affiliation (3) information gathering (4) religion, and (5) optimism (Dimsdale, 1982). Insofar as any of these coping mechanisms are successful, we can play a role in fostering them in a patient. We also find maladaptive mechanisms indicative of some failure to cope, such as social isolation, extreme anxiety with exacerbation of pain, and passive dependency. Again, the variety of helpers in the health care system can be mutually supportive for individual patients, and the physical therapist can play a vital, active role in promoting appropriate adaptation to pain.

COMPONENTS OF PAIN

The complexity of pain explains why it is difficult to treat. The range of types of pain appears to us in a spectrum from purely organic pain to purely psychogenic in nature. Organic pain may be felt at the site of primary stimulation, or felt at a site other than that of original stimulation but in tissues supplied by the same or adjacent neural segments—this is known as referred pain. In addition, somatic pain can be due to reflex adaptive mechanisms to an original noxious stimulation, such as pain generated by muscle splinting which creates a new source of noxious impulse.

Psychogenic origins of pain may be explained in terms of the meaning which pain has to an individual. For some, there are links between pain, evil and sin, and pain may be a necessary form of guilt and punishment, essential for the individual's psychological equilibrium (Degenaar, 1979). But for most people in pain, there is a combination, to varying degrees, of somatic and psychogenic origins. A patient's past experiences play a role in his total experience of pain, as does his culture and his emotional make-up. Clinical challenges may help us to formulate some basic questions about these complex components of pain. Can we integrate psychic pain with neurophysiologic theories of pain or neuro-hormonal theories? If we try, does it help us decide how to treat pain?

THEORIES OF PAIN

A very brief review of the more prominent theories of pain may prove useful to the reader of this volume who faces clinical decision-making every day and who may seek some insights from these various authors.

Neurophysiologic pain theories

Specificity theory of Von Frey (Von Frey, 1894)

This theory was one of the first efforts to develop a coherent physiologic theory of pain. It states that there are four cutaneous sensory modalities: touch, warmth, cold, pain. Each sense is carried on a specific nerve fiber pathway. Pain impulses are carried from free nerve endings scattered widely throughout the skin, subcutaneous tissues and viscera. The neural paths are made up of small, unmyelinated C fibers which travel either through nerve trunks to the posterior roots of the spinal cord or through sympathetic nerve trunks to sympathetic ganglia and on to posterior roots of the spinal cord. Thus, discrete pain pathways exist which carry pain-sense from the central nervous system to specific centers (like a telephone network). Some of the neurosurgical techniques which have evolved are based on this theory, such as nerve blocks, tractotomies, sympathectomies, posterior rhizotomies and cordotomies.

Two pathway theory of Head (Head et al, 1905)

This refinement of the original specificity theory was necessary when two different types and sizes of nerve fibers were discovered to be involved in pain transmission: A delta epsilon fibers and C fibers. Each pathway was responsible for a different and unique pain sensation. The A delta epsilon system was termed the epicritic pain pathway, responsible for a sharp, pricking type of pain, carried via the lateral spinothalamic tract in the neospinothalamic division, involving the reticular activating system. The slower C fibers carried a burning type of pain called protopathic, which became more severe when stimulation of this pathway became repetitive, due to summation. This pathway is carried on the ventral spinothalamic tract in the paleo-division. With this elaboration of neuroanatomy and physiology, neurosurgeons could become more precise in their techniques for pain alleviation.

Pattern theory (Weddell et al, 1948)

According to this theory, there are no specific pain pathways or nerve endings, as refuted by the following pieces of evidence. (1) Both noxious and non-noxious stimulation can lead to pain. Warmth can lead to hot which goes on in intensity to pain. This is true of cold, pressure, and other forms of non-painful stimulation. (2) Pain can occur long after a noxious stimulation is withdrawn, that is, after a delay. (3) Psychiatric evidence for painful experience refutes a simple pathway theory. (4) C fiber free nerve endings also carry impulses for other sensations, and not only for pain. The sensation of pain does not depend upon one pathway or two, but upon the total central projection along all existing pathways of all the impulses coming into the central nervous system pain reception area. Pain perception is due to the stimulus intensity and spatial and temporal summation of all impulses, such that when there is a hyper-synchronization of impulse volleys impinging at once, pain is interpreted.

Reverberating circuits (Livingston, 1943; Inman, 1968)

A specific case of the pattern theory, this theory attempts to explain such central phenomena as causalgia and phantom pain. This describes a central patterning of impulse flow, which creates for the patient a 'painful memory'. There is no peripheral stimulus, which has been withdrawn by an amputation or by healing of a peripheral nerve injury. Instead, a fixed pattern is locked into the central structures because it cannot be modified, as there is no normal sensory input from the original source possible.

Gate control theory (Melzack & Wall, 1965)

This very widely believed theory is an extension of the pattern theory. Pain perception is the result of central and peripheral inputs, both of which act upon a 'gate' which controls the transmission of impulses to the pain centers of the thalamus and cerebral cortex. The gate is located in a portion of the dorsal column of the spinal cord at each segmental level, called the substantia gelatinosa. Peripheral input to the gate is comprised of two types, one mediated on large size A fibers, the other on small C fibers. It is the combined influence of both inputs which influences the gate. To open this gate to pain perception, a predominance of C fiber input must prevail. Dominance is established by impulse traffic and by spatial and temporal summation at the level of the gate. To close the gate to pain, A fiber input must predominate. A sized fibers carry touch, pressure, and thermal stimuli, while C fibers carry cutaneous 'pain' and cold. Sustained impulses from large type A fibers inhibit transmission of pain to central cells. These peripheral impulses are always subject to modification by emotion, experience (memory) and other cortical functions.

Non-neurophysiologic pain theories

Behavioralist theory (Fordyce, 1973)

A behavioralist approach to chronic pain is based upon the conception that 'pain behaviors', such as grimacing, clutching a painful part, popping a pain pill, moaning or crying, or stopping all activity, are all used to communicate pain. These types of behaviors usually bring results, such as sympathy from family, rest from activity with some relief of pain and more attention paid to the person displaying these. Thus, the behaviours themselves can become rewarding and inherently satisfying. If these behaviors are reinforced more than 'well behaviors' it is likely that a person would learn to display pain behavior even when there was no longer an active pathogenic factor causing pain. The physical therapist who directs his patient with chronic pain to lift weights until he feels pain but then to stop, is reinforcing the stopping of exercise, a form of pain behavior, and promotes the repetition of this behavior. The same patient learns from his therapist that it is better to stop exercise, i.e. not exercise at all perhaps, than to experience any pain with exercise. Total avoidance of motion can easily result from this interpretation. The treatment approach used by the behavioralist is to ignore pain behaviors in order to extinguish them or at least to not reinforce them. An exercise program is set up with regular intervals of rest and motion, regardless of pain, but to be safe, the intervals are set to avoid pain as much as possible. The Pain Clinic idea, as described in Chapter 10, explains in much greater detail the usefulness of the behavioralist theory on many dimensions of treatment.

Endogenous opiate theory (Werle, 1972)

Among the newer theories based upon biochemical substances found in the nervous system, this theory could be classed a neurophysiologic one, but it differs from older ones by not describing neuron pathways. Instead, it relates the discovery of two types of neurotransmitters, the enkephalins, small peptide molecules, and β-endorphin, a large peptide involving long sequencing of amino acids, to pain sensation and adaptation. According to this discovery the body manufactures opiate-like substances in order to provide pain relief at specific receptor-sites in the central nervous system. These substances are similar in effect to morphine, and react at receptor-sites to inactivate pain sensation. Enkephalins are found in the caudate nucleus, the anterior hypothalamus, and the substantia gelatinosa, and because of their relatively simple structure, have a rapid-acting effect which terminates in about 2 minutes. The β-endorphin is found in the pituitary gland and has a 4 hour or longer effect. It takes a larger pain or stress stimulus to generate the β-endorphin response than it does to activate the enkephalin response. It is postulated that these substances, like morphine, can become addictive, but as endogenous substances, the result of the addiction may be seen as the seeking of specific stress or pain-generating conditions. The example cited most often is the exercise fanatic who chooses to exercise for very long periods on a daily basis at rather high levels of stress. It may be true that the person with chronic or intractable pain is 'addicted' to his pain through this mechanism, and that although the role of these substances is pain alleviation, the interpretation by such patients is the inappropriate one of continued pain.

Perhaps it is clear to the reader that there is nonrefutable evidence for many of these theories of pain, and that although they are treated as distinct, mutually exclusive theories, the whole truth must incorporate aspects of nearly all of them. How to interweave the theories is not at all clear, and much more research in the basic physiology of pain is needed to provide the full fabric to our understanding of pain. As previously stated, each approach provides for its believers a language of pain, generating the narrower view of what pain must be, and thus, of how to evaluate and treat it.

RATIONALE FOR TREATMENT OF PAIN

The narrow view of pain most probably leaves out dimensions which are likely to be important to treatment of a specific patient. Whichever theory seems to be the model of best fit for this patient is the one used to provide the rationale for treatment. Or, whichever theory fits best with the treatment approach the physical therapist or physician or psychologist is most familiar or comfortable with, is the one chosen to provide the rationale. Thus, the neuro-surgeon subscribes to the specific pathway theory, and the person administering transcutaneous nerve stimulation bases his therapy on the Gate Control Theory. An acupuncture therapy has been vari-ously explained by the gate control theory (Rozier, 1974) and the endogenous opiate theory (Nathan, 1978). The notion of psycho-therapy for pain treatment fits into a 'Pain as a determinant of the quality of our consciousness' framework, a more psychological, even philosophical point of view (Degenaar, 1979).

A more important rationale is provided, not by pain theories, but by our own initial evaluation of our patient. The medical diagnosis which provides us with the pathogenic mechanism for the pain, or our own findings, will suggest restorative treatment approaches to use in the type of condition which is acute, reversible and of clear etiology. Thus, pain generated by edema suggests several treatments to reduce edema, and pain caused by tightness of specific muscles suggests a variety of treatments available to relieve muscle tightness. More difficult cases are those whose pain is chronic and of uncertain or untreatable cause. Now we imagine a rationale for treatment as supportive or helping a patient control pain. The post-herpetic type of pain appears to be of this nature, and certain treatment tech-niques can be useful in controlling the pain experienced. Certain types of pain from cancer should not be approached in the same way as pain for which restorative or supportive treatments are in-dicated. In this case, palliative treatments may have the most ap-propriate rationale, and it may make the most sense to explore with each patient the best form of palliative treatment for him.

From the point of view of finding the best, most appropriate ra-tionale for treatment, each patient case must be considered in de-tail. This point brings out how absolutely vital pre-treatment assessments are. As the contributors to this volume demonstrate, pain assessment is only a small part of the total evaluation of the patient who needs treatment for pain. If restorative therapy is ap-propriate, then pain measurement is a small part of a much bigger evaluation package to determine the processes which can be re-versed. Pain per se is one of several indexes to indicate effectiveness of treatment. If supportive therapy is indicated, pain measurement is necessary to set the baseline initially and to judge effectiveness of any approach taken. Other evaluations may be helpful to decide upon one therapeutic procedure capable of producing the desired effect. However, pain measurement will provide the most direct index. In palliative treatment, the major evaluation may well be the patient's personal experience of pain and relief from pain. Since pain measurement contributes a diverse set of information, it is a useful fact that there exists such a wide variety of methods to measure pain or different aspects of pain.

MEASUREMENT

Pain intensity is a measurement based upon the sensory component of pain alone and has been measured using scales with rankings in numbers or in word descriptors. But because words have different meanings for different people and for one person over time, and therefore have no universal anchorage, these scales are often not reliable over time. Several techniques of sensory matching have been developed to avoid this problem. In these techniques, some alternate sense or pain experience is used to create an analogue of the clinical pain. One such technique is the use of an audiometer in which the decibel signal being heard by the patient is matched to the intensity of the pain being experienced (Peck, 1967). Another method is the ischemic tourniquet test in which degrees of ischemic pain, as measured by *duration* of ischemia created by a tourniquet at a constant pressure, are matched to the intensity of clinical pain (Sternbach et al, 1977).

But pain measurement must go beyond intensity for most clinical uses, especially as we try to account for the emotional, distressful component to pain. Qualitative measures have also been made available to us for this purpose. The most widely used measure of this type is the McGill-Melzack Questionnaire, printed in this volume as its use is described by several authors. In this questionnaire, many words are suggested for selection by the person in pain, and word categories help us to analyze the distress component of the pain.

Additional approaches to the measurement of pain need to be explored. In the psychiatric setting, the fascinating method described in Chapter 2, called the GPM method of evaluation, offers new insights which could be adapted to other clinical settings. As the reader reads on in this volume, the issue of pain measurement is dealt with in many different ways by the authors describing different treatment approaches. Perhaps one treatment approach lends itself better to one pain measurement technique, or perhaps clinicians gain access and then skill in applying one measure of pain for all patients? It seems worthwhile to explore several measures in order to determine the validity of each, approapriateness for the clinical problem or type of pain, accuracy, and reliability. Then the measurement results could be used more rationally for the selection of the most appropriate form of treatment for each individual patient.

TREATMENT

There are many worthwhile forms of treatment for pain, many of which are represented by chapters in this volume. Notably missing are discussions of the more conventional, perhaps old-fashioned treatments still being widely applied and still bringing good clinical results to many patients. Examples of these forms of treatment are: massage, traction, heat, cold, bracing, specific exercise approaches. Also missing in this volume are chapters on some little known, much less conventional treatment methods, such as laser therapy, reflex approaches (Van Stralen, 1982) and Chinese 'Shi Kung' (Zhuo et al, 1983). Although new approaches and new clinical theories to back them are essential additions to the profession of physical therapy, each new contribution must be subjected to rigorous theoretical and practical tests before it is applied to the vast population of pain patients. If they are simply presented and applied and accepted on the basis that 'they work' because pain patients report subjective relief, then we are practicing witch-craft and will not gain credibility in the realm of the wider practice of medicine. Furthermore, we are breaching the sacred trust and jeopardizing the health and safety of our patients on whom untested methods are applied. The reader will note that each of the approaches described here have been studied to some large degree in controlled trials, many conducted by these same authors. Bibliographic materials have been included to allow readers to become more familiar with both the type of scientific testing done for these methods, and also with the gaps still existing where further tests are needed. At the end of this volume is the annotated bibliography, presented in topics and by country, to help the reader select more extensive readings for a more complete review.

Many of our more conventional physical therapy treatment measures have not been subjected to the type of scientific inquiry necessary today, yet are widely used and believed in. Presumably, these have not been harmful to the majority of our patients, but without the sort of careful study of their comparative effects they cannot be applied in the most rational manner but rather in a somewhat random way. This means that although patients get better or feel better temporarily in association with their treatment, we have no way of knowing what really brought relief, or a cure. The cause and effect relationship is easily assumed but may be entirely erroneous, as it is, for example, when you push a light button just at the moment when the whole city of New York experiences a black-out. The advantage of having the information needed to establish cause and effect and dose-response relationships for each of our treatments, is that we may then apply each therapeutic intervention in precisely the appropriate dosage (intensity, frequency, duration, mode) to achieve a maximum benefit in the least period of time. We can also study the additive effects of several interventions including inter-actions with pain drugs; for example, exercise parameters appro-priate under the influence of narcotic-sedative drug therapy. The effect of any one treatment upon all systems necessary to normal function, and not only upon the pain itself, should be investigated. Each form of treatment presents as a stimulus (sometimes simple, as in electrotherapy, or sometimes complex, as in exercise or mass-age) which produces patterns of response in the nervous system, both somatic and autonomic, in the circulatory, respiratory, mus-culoskeletal, and neurohumeral systems. Responses in one system will inevitably influence reponses in all the other systems and result in changes which may effect the experience of pain. Due to the complexities of the human body as a responsive organism, many more careful studies of stimulus-response need to be undertaken, and should be conducted by the physical therapist who imposes the stimuli therapeutically and studies the responses at least in terms of the patient's subjective complaints. Improving our objective means of studying these responses will lend us greater depth of understanding of our treatment effects.

The series of questions a clinician should ask while making the decision about which treatment to apply to a specific patient's pain, which leads her to study objectively the intervention applied, the responses to it and the results from it are as follows:

1. What is the nature of my stimulus? What are its dimensions, the dosage of the stimulus?
2. What structure is sensitive to the stimulus I am giving?
3. What function am I trying to influence?
4. Are some of the several effects of the stimulus in conflict with the specific therapeutic goals? Or with other goals of the same treatment?
5. Has the pathological state altered the system which is relied

upon to produce healing from pain? Or has it placed on altered demand upon the healing system?

6. Is the pathology in the healing system, or is it affecting it from outside?

7. If I plan to use two or more modalities, what is my net gain going to be? How have I changed the relationship between the two modalities by preceding one with the other?

8. Can I use a modality in such a way that I can be more selective in a response?

9. How can I determine the adequacy of the neural reflex arc which will be required to work in a particular patient, using a particular stimulus?

As implied by these nine questions, each treatment can be, and should be, the subject of a scientific study, and can be handled as a valuable information-gathering experiment, so that over time such data are pooled and new insight can be gleaned from each experience with patients. Although this process sounds time-consuming and therefore clinically unfeasible, what I am advocating is *not* spending more time with each patient, but, rather, having more objective means of evaluating responses and varying the input of stimuli in more systematic ways. Since therapists do consider it important to evaluate patients before, during and after treatment, the time spent doing this is presumably already budgeted and should be used to better advantage.

To summarize, I believe that we physical therapists have made three errors in the way we have gone about selecting appropriate treatment for our patients. First, we have looked at the effect of a stimulus on one function at a time, yet we may actually be effecting more than one variable at once. Second, we have assumed that the stimulus modality we have used has altered a function in only one direction. We must take ample measurements to determine the response pattern and be prepared for the possibility of a paradoxical response. Third, we have maintained an oversimplified concept of a disease pattern or a pain pattern, assuming a causative agent. We need more generalized concepts to transfer our knowledge of the responses of one patient to the next.

CONTRIBUTIONS TO THIS VOLUME

Following this introductory chapter, the reader will find two somewhat general topics, both of which also deal with specific points on evaluation and treatment and present case examples. The first of these is the only chapter dedicated to evaluation, and presents quite a unique form of evaluation now in use in parts of Norway. The second of these reviews the psychology of pain and describes the physical therapist in a psychologist's role in dealing with the whole patient. Specific treatment approaches are also brought in.

The next two chapters discuss two well-known and well-documented treatment approaches, that of transcutaneous electrical nerve stimulation (TENS) and acupuncture. Of the two, acupuncture is perhaps less accessible to the clinician because its use involves extra training. However, it can be found in use increasingly throughout the world, especially in the Orient where it originated.

Chapters 6 and 7 both describe manual therapy, but from two different viewpoints. Manipulation of joints and techniques of manual therapy are widely used in the West and Australia for orthopaedic clinical problems, but within the specialty area controversies about when to use and how to use techniques exist. These two papers show agreement on many aspects, but disagree on others, thus highlighting differing points of view and areas where further research may be necessary to clear up controversial issues.

The next chapter deals with a very special pain problem, and one extremely difficult to treat: the painful hemiplegic shoulder. The Candian author's experience and research with this clinical problem using EMG biofeedback provides valuable insights for other clinicians tackling the same problem.

Finally, two chapters on a more interdisciplinary and global approach to pain control are presented: the Swedish Back School experience, emphasizing education and fitness, and ergonomic assessment; and the Pain Clinic approach found widely in the U.S.A. and British Commonwealth. The Mississippi pain clinic may be unique in one major regard, which is that the physical therapist is a co-director of the clinic and as such plays a major role in the patient's total experience of residing in such a clinic.

At the very end of this volume is the Annotated Bibliography, where references selected by these authors and a few added knowledgeable people are provided with paragraphs describing briefly their contents. This bibliography should give you, the reader, some idea of the usefulness of these articles to you in your own particular setting so that you can acquire for your further study any which from this list appear to have significance for you.

My own hope is that by reading this volume clinicians who see pain patients daily will begin to see the importance of rigorous clini-

cal trials on treatment and responses to treatment, and follow it up
with efforts to engage in the types of research necessary to further
the development of our profession and establish the efficacy of our
own therapeutic efforts on behalf of these, often difficult, pain
problems.

REFERENCES

Degenaar J J 1979 Some philosophical considerations on pain. Pain 7: 281–304
Dimsdale J 1982 Helping patients cope. Consultant July: 171–180
Fordyce W E 1973 An operant conditioning method for managing chronic pain.
    Post-graduate Medicine 53:123
Head H, Rivers W, Sherren J 1905 The afferent nervous system from a new
    aspect. Brain 28:99
Inman V T 1968 Clinical pathologic consideration of pain mechanism: New
    concepts. In: Pain and its clinical management. F A Davis Co., Philadelphia
Johnson M 1977 Assessment of clinical pain. In: Jacox A K (ed) Pain: a source
    book for nurses and other health professionals. Little Brown & Co, Boston,
    pp 139–166
Livingston W K 1943 Pain mechanisms: a physiologic interpretation of causalgia
    and its related states. MacMillan, New York
Melzack R, Wall P D 1965 Pain mechanisms: a new theory. Science 150: 971–979
Nathan P W 1978 Acupuncture analgesia. Trends in Neurosciences 1(1): 21–23
Peck R 1967 A precise technique for the measurement of pain. Headache
    6: 189–194
Rozier C K 1974 Acupuncture for pain relief. Physical Therapy 54(9): 949–952
Sternbach R A 1974 Pain patients: traits and treatment. Academic Press, New
    York
Sternbach R A, Deems L M, Timmermans G, Huey L Y 1977 On the sensitivity
    of the tourniquet pain test. Pain 3: 105–110
Van Stralen C 1982 Somatosympathetic reflex activity in segmental therapy.
    Proceedings from the IX International Congress for Physical Therapy.
    Stockholm, Sweden, pp 299–304
Von Frey M 1894 Die Gefühle und ihr Verhältnis zu den Empfindungen. Beit. z.
    Physiol. des Schmerzsinnes. Berichte über die verhandlung d. königl. sächs.
    Gesellschaft d. Wissenschaften, Leipzig
Werle E 1972 On endogenous producing substances with particular reference to
    plasmakinins. In: Janzen R, Keidel W D, Herz A, Steichele C, Payne J P,
    Burt R A P (eds) Pain. William & Wilkins Co, Baltimore
Zhuo D, Dighe J, Basmajian J V 1983 EMG biofeedback and Chinese 'Chi
    Kung': relaxation effects in patients with low back pain. Physiotherapy Canada
    35(1): 13–18

Muscular pains and psychopathology: evaluation by the GPM method

The patient referred to physical therapy with the complaint of sore or painful muscles represents a professional challenge in the process of evaluation and treatment. One common pitfall may be to over-look the muscular status of the entire body and to concentrate only upon the part of the body which the patient spontanously reports as painful. The localized muscular pain is an important sign of dys-function, but diagnosis of the cause of pain may be difficult.

It is important to examine the condition of the muscles of the entire body of the patient with local pains since there is a close re-lationship between the skeletal muscular system, the psychological defense mechanisms and psychopathological conditions. The objec-tives of this paper are to demonstrate:

— The use of the Global Physiotherapeutic Muscle Examination (GPM) in evaluating patients with muscular pains
— The importance of using all palpatable pains throughout the body as a clue in treatment planning
— The method of integrating the GPM results with the patient's somatic and psychological symptoms, social functioning and life situation in treatment planning.

MUSCULAR PAINS AND PSYCHOPATHOLOGY

It is common knowledge that muscular pains may be a symptom of an acute or chronic nervous disorder (Braatoy, 1954; Reich, 1950; Lowen, 1958). A person in a stressful life situation will begin to automatically strengthen his defenses by 'pulling himself to-gether' both muscularly and psychologically. This tightening of muscles may alter the physiological condition of the skeletal mus-cles, and sooner or later some of these muscles may be felt as painful.

In spite of a rather general tightening of the muscles in many parts of the body, the pains are usually localized only to some mus-

cle groups. Which group of muscles will be the first to be felt as painful, seems to depend upon several factors:
— If some muscles were tighter than others before the actual stressful situation started, these muscles will often be those which are first felt as painful when they are tightened even more.
— Previous muscular trauma, overwork or skeletal dysfunctions, may make certain muscle groups more vulnerable to developing a painful response in stress situations.
— Some muscle groups may be actively involved in the inhibition of certain (forbidden) feelings. The muscles of the jaw and the shoulders/arms seem, for instance, to be closely related to the inhibition and repression of aggressive feelings (Heiberg, 1980).

The palpation of muscle throughout the entire body will commonly reveal painful muscles of which the patient was previously unaware. The interpretation of this phenomenon is still not fully understood. Clinical experience has, however, shown that such muscles may be viewed as latently painful muscles. If one tries to eliminate local pains in one region, some of these latent painful muscular pains which caused the patient to seek treatment are a sign frequency of pains in muscles, both daily pains and pains on palpation, may be seen as an indication of the degree of actual psychological stress which the patient tries to cope with. If the localized muscular pains which caused the patient to seek treatment are a sign of a higher than normal muscle activity, or a sign of a person being in a too stressful life situation, localized treatment directed only towards alleviating the locally painful region may result in:
— No change—the pains are unchanged.
— The pains disappear, but other muscular parts of the body become painful instead.
— The pains disappear, but recur within a short period of time.

In addition to these three outcomes, another possible outcome which is significant is: the muscular pains may disappear, but the patient gets more nervous. He may become more depressed, more anxious, more restless or dizzy, sometimes to a degree that necessitates psychiatric hospitalization (Karterud, 1980). Such reactions demonstrate the close connection between the tightened painful muscles and the psychological defense mechanism. If through therapeutic intervention an effort is made to relax the locally tight muscles and thereby loosen up the psychological defenses more than the patient is able to tolerate, several unwanted consequences may be the result:
— The patient may unconsciously manage to resist relaxation of

the painful muscles, and the pain will continue or get worse.
— A tightness and rigidity of other muscle groups may develop to compensate for the reduction of the emotional defense in the treated muscles and newly involved muscle groups will be felt as painful instead. These two reactions are most common among patients exhibiting a relatively strong ego and neurotic behaviour.
— Patients with a certain degree of ego weakness, patients on the edge of a nervous breakdown or psychosis may not tolerate relaxation therapy. The painful muscles may represent their last line of defense. In these patients the other muscles of the body may not be able to take over when the physical therapist manages to relax the painful muscles. The relaxation therapy, when inappropriately applied, can precipitate the patient developing a nervous breakdown and/or psychosis. A physical therapist who is considering the use of relaxation therapy with ego-weak patients, should work closely with a psychiatrist and/or psychotherapist to avoid a potentially destructive outcome of the therapy (Houge, 1978). It is, therefore, important that the physical therapist is able to assess both the muscular and the psychological resources of a patient.

NECESSARY CHARACTERISTICS OF AN EVALUATION OF MUSCLE STATUS.

How do we evaluate a patient with muscular pains? It should be obvious that we need an examination which fulfills the following criteria:
1. It should be useful and applicable in daily clinical work.
2. It should be reliable, i.e. if two or more physical therapists examine the same patient, their findings should be similar.
3. It should be valid, i.e. one examines the property one intends to measure.
4. It should give detailed information of the deviations of a single muscle, of different muscle groups and of the general muscular status of the entire body.
5. It should describe valid information about the patient's possible degree of psychopathology based on the gathered data of different single muscle examinations throughout the entire body and the general muscle status.
6. Together with the knowledge of the patient's life situation, social

functioning and mental health, it should also give sufficient information for rational treatment planning.

The Global Physiotherapeutic Examination has been developed by Sundsvold 1966–73 (Sundsvold, 1969, 1975, 1976) based on the earlier work of physical therapist Bülow-Hansen (1967) and other physical therapists. After Sundsvold's cooperation with Vaglum started in 1973, the GPM has been further refined and tested for validity and reliability. Denstad has also given a valuable contribution to this work. A book containing a detailed description of the GPM and with pictures of every single examination is published in Norwegian (Sundsvold et al, 1982).

GPM has for several years been used both in the routine clinical work and in research, and has fulfilled the necessary characteristics of a physical therapy evaluation. We will first briefly describe the main principles of the GPM, its reliability and its use in evaluating the degree of psychopathology. Thereafter, we will present two cases, one with low back pain and one with chest pain, which illustrate the use of the GPM in evaluation and treatment planning.

THE GPM METHOD

The GPM is a somatic examination which gives information about muscular status throughout the entire body and some aspects of the mental health of the patient, i.e. the possible degree of psychopathology. Three versions of the GPM exist. The large version consists of 313 variables that are tested, a medium version of GPM of 184 variables and a short version of 72 variables. The medium version is a selection of variables abstracted from the large version. In the medium version, only the left side of the body is tested, in addition to all non-side-specific tests.

The short version is used in this paper. It is abstracted from the medium version. The variables were selected based on two criteria:
— to get an equal distribution of variables throughout the entire body and from each of the 12 categories of examination
— based on the findings of four separate research projects, variables were selected which had the greatest capacity for discriminating between groups of patients with different degrees of psychopathology.

Because of this selection of variables, it is possible to use the total sum score of the short version to evaluate the degree (not type) of psychopathology in individual patients. For treatment planning, the data collected by the short version of the GPM may occasionally need to be supplemented with variables from the large version of GPM and/or more specific physical therapy musculoskeletal assessment. The examination using the short version takes approximately 30 minutes, and the large version takes about 90 minutes.

Carrying out the GPM

The examination is carried out in private with only the physical therapist and the patient present, and in one session. The patient should be dressed in shorts and a halter top. Before initiating the examination, the patient is told that he will receive a verbal summary of the findings following completion of the examination. The physical therapist starts the examination by introducing herself and explaining procedures involved in the examination. The patient is asked to report what he is feeling during the examination and is told that he may ask for a pause at any time. Detailed information about the case history and social functioning should be taken afterwards. Each new step in the examination is carefully explained before it is carried out. At intervals the patient is asked to relax. He should not be exposed to surprises and should all the time feel safe and have a good rapport with the physical therapist. Talking should be limited and only related to the examination because both the physical therapist and the patient need to concentrate on the examination. The patient should leave the GPM examination with a feeling of being met with respect and adequately taken care of. The first meeting with the physical therapist is of crucial importance for giving the patient a positive feeling and contact with his own body, and also for building up a good patient–therapist relationship for possible future treatment.

Twelve GPM categories

To get as comprehensive a description as possible of muscle status throughout the body, the GPM consists of twelve different categories of examination. Each category examines different aspects of muscle status and properties of the muscle (for example, standing position, respiration, passive gravity movements, etc.). Each category examines the same muscle characteristics. In the short version, each category consists of six variables distributed throughout the entire body.

The twelve categories are:

Inspection of postures

1. Standing position. (Gives information about the postural muscles and the stretch reflex.)
2. Lying supine. (Gives information related to changes in muscle contraction with changes in posture and other muscles (normally not involved) which are activated in supine position.)
3. Other positions: the maximal extent of passive range of movement. (Gives information about joint range and the general joint muscle status.)

Inspection of respiration

4. Degree of the amplitude of inspiration on five different places of the front trunk, rhythm and frequency in standing position. (Gives information about the muscles of respiration and the autonomic nervous system.)
5. Degree of the amplitude of inspiration on five different places of the front trunk, rhythm and frequency in supine position. (Gives information about the muscles of respiration and the autonomic nervous system.)

Evaluation of movements

6. The resistance to passive movements against the force of gravity when the body is already in a resting position. (Gives information about muscle tension.)
7. The resistance to passive movements. (Gives information about muscle tension.)
8. The maximal extent of active range of movement. (Gives information about muscle tension and the general joint muscle status.)

The three types of movements give information about different qualities of muscle tension.

Evaluation by palpation

The palpation is done in the lying position while the patient is asked to relax, thus preventing movements in the muscle. Our clinical hypothesis is that palpation of the muscles under such circumstances estimates physiological muscle properties, not tonus. Aiken (1980) referring to Basmajian (1978) also says that neurophysiologists now generally agree that in a completely relaxed muscle (as by the GPM palpation) no neuro-muscular activity is present. This may be the reason why we found no correlation between EMG findings and the palpation findings in a small pilot study in 1974. More physiological research is needed to clarify exactly the physiological characteristics of the muscles assessed by palpation. Our hypothesis is that by specific palpation techniques it is possible to assess deviations in the connective tissue and the amount of fluid in the muscles:

9. Stretch palpation: stretching of connective tissue and muscle fibers across the muscle belly. The direction of stretch is across the longitudinal axis of the muscle. (Gives physiological information about the stretchability of the connective tissue and the muscle fibers.)

10. Press palpation: pressing together the muscle belly; the bundles in the muscle, the muscle fibers and the fluid in the muscle, applying a press grip across the muscle belly and compressing the fluid, the muscle fibers and the bundles in the muscle. (Gives information about the amount of fluid (circulation) in the muscle.)

11. The patient's subjective reaction to stretch palpation in one muscle. (Gives information from the sensory system.)

12. The press palpation of the skin. (Gives information about the circulation in the skin.)

Examining the subjective reactions to stretch palpation (palpational pain)

Since the topic of this book is pain, we will describe in more detail the examination of the subjective reaction to stretch palpation. This is recorded in lying supine when each muscle is stretch palpated. When palpated, some patients spontaneously tell what they experience or feel, some do not. To ensure more systematic and comparable information from patient to patient, in the GPM one records the subjective reactions to every stretch palpation on a 12 point scale, going from neutral, indifferent reactions, over to pleasant, good, good but painful, and to unpleasant and sickening. Before starting the palpation, the patient gets the following instruction: 'You will need to cooperate when I am examining your muscles. Each time I am stretching your muscle I want you to tell me how you experience it. You may for instance feel it is pleasant, comfortable or have a more neutral/indifferent reaction. If you feel it is uncomfortable, you may describe it as sore, unpleasant or sickening. You may also have other feelings.' The task of the physical therapist is to give the patient freedom to express whatever he feels, and to help with the use of simple non-leading questions to categorize the answers and place them on the rating scale. An example may illustrate the procedure:

The physical therapist stretch palpates musculus tibialis anterior and asks the patient: 'What do you feel here?'
Patient: 'It hurts. It reminds me of a hurdle race when I was a school boy.'
Physical therapist: 'Do you like to think of that race, or do you associate it with something unpleasant?
Patient: 'I stumbled and hurt that muscle in the race. I had pains in it for a long time. Now it is unpleasant when you grasp the muscle.'
Physical therapist: 'Do you think it is a little unpleasant or more sickening when I stretch it?'
Patient: 'It is really sickening.'

As to the interpretation of these palpation pains, we have earlier mentioned that such muscles may be viewed as latently painful muscles. Clinical experience indicates that a high frequency of painful muscles by stretch palpation may indicate that the patient is in a stressful life situation which he tries to cope with by tightening his muscles and thereby strengthening his psychological defences at the same time. A high frequency of painful reactions and a high frequency of indifferent reactions may also tell something about the patient's relationship to his own body. In a small study (Sundsvold & Vaglum, 1982), it was found that borderline patients (Gunderson & Singer, 1975) had significantly more often indifferent reactions than a group of ego weak neurotic patients. Borderline patients are characterized by an identity diffusion, and they will also often report their depressive state as a kind of emptiness. There appears to be a parallel between the identity diffusion and feelings of emptiness on one hand and a relative lack of sensitivity when their muscles are stretch palpated on the other. As to the painful reactions to stretch palpation, we found in our studies that the psychiatric inpatients significantly had the most deviant reactions, next came the patients in a private physical therapy office and lastly the healthy control people (Sundsvold et al, 1975).

Recording the findings from the GPM examination of individual patients

Single tests

The findings of every single test is recorded by use of a predefined 12 point numerical scale. Each score indicates the degree of deviation from an empirically defined ideal muscle condition. The deviation can go in two directions: (a) less than ideal response (negative scores), (b) more than ideal response (positive scores). According to this, the scales are constructed in such a way that the ideal condition gets the score 0, while positive or negative scores are indicated on each side of the ideal condition.

Computing sum scores of the twelve categories

Results from the single examinations in the twelve categories of the short version of the GPM are summarized into twelve sum scores in the following way. The physical therapist summarizes each negative and each positive score from all the single examinations into a negative (less than ideal response) and a positive (more than ideal response) sum score. The negative and positive values of the sum scores are then marked on the scales for each of the twelve categories as shown in the form in Figure 2.1. The 0-line in the middle indicates the ideal condition (value 0), the sum scores of the negative deviations are marked to the left, and the sum scores of the positive deviations are marked to the right.

By drawing lines between the marks on the 12 scales, one gets a profile or pattern of the findings describing each patient's overall muscle status. The physical therapist can easily see where the patient has his muscular resources and deficiencies. In Figure 2.1, the two dotted lines on both sides of the 0-line illustrate the sum score from a healthy person with minor muscular deviations, and the two solid lines illustrate the GPM findings from a psychotic inpatient. The psychotic inpatient has many more deviant findings than the healthy person in this case, especially in his reactions to stretch palpation (palpational pains). He also shows major distortions in the ability to perform passive gravity movements, in the range of passive motion and in the respiration findings. Some of the negative sum scores are also too big, especially the pressure palpation findings. This shows that this psychotic patient is a very flexed, tight and inhibited person and that the muscles and skin feel

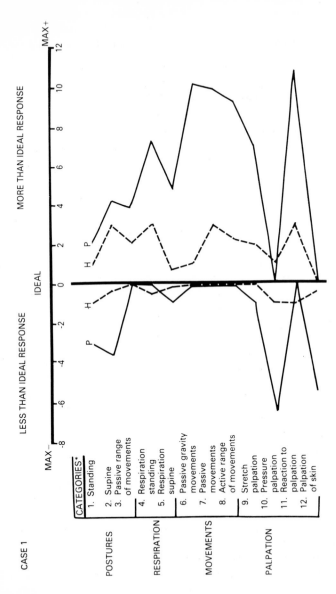

MUSCULAR PAINS AND PSYCHOPATHOLOGY 27

Fig. 2.1 The sumscores of 12 categories in the GPM-examination showing the muscle pattern of a healthy person — H (dotted lines) and a psychotic inpatient — P (solid lines)

GPM total sumscore of the healthy person = 28 and of the psychotic person = 90.
*Sumscore of 6 separate assessments in each category.

dry. Clinically, the form in Figure 2.1 is only used to plot the muscle findings for one patient, but here the results for two patients are plotted to allow a comparison. If the findings are recorded at the beginning and at the end of a treatment, one can easily see in what ways and to what degree that patient's muscular pattern has changed.

Total sum score (short version)

The next step in evaluation is to summarize all the sum scores from the twelve categories into a negative and a positive total sum score. Lastly are summarized the total negative and the total positive sum scores, without regard to negative and positive signs, into the total sum score. The total sum score indicates the degree of muscular deviation throughout the body which the patient has at the present time. This total sum score also gives indications about the degree of psychopathology. We will come back to this later.

RELIABILITY

A useful clinical assessment tool must be reliable. If two physical therapists examine the same patient, they should arrive at nearly the same conclusion. The lack of a reliable muscular examination method has made research difficult in physical therapy. The GPM method has been shown to have a sufficient potential reliability, and a brief description of findings from an inter-tester reliability study (Sundsvold et al, 1982) will be included.

The reliability study of a 50-variable version of the GPM consisting of single variables from all 12 categories was carried out by letting 3 physical therapists (A, B and C) independently examine 25 persons (11 psychiatric inpatients and 14 staff members) without knowing the findings from the other therapists. Physical therapist A was one of the authors of this paper (M.Ø.S.) and has developed the GPM. B had used the GPM method for several years, while C had used it only for a short time and never for research purposes. Before the study, the physical therapists trained for 12 hours over a period of one month examining the same people. The inter-tester correlations (Pearsons r) between the total sum scores of two and two physical therapists were: $r_{AB} = 0.89$, $r_{AC} = 0.90$, $r_{BC} = 0.83$. This shows a sufficient consensus about ranking of the people on the basis of total muscular deviations. On the basis of the correlation coefficients, we have also computed the reliability coefficient

R for each physical therapist (see Fleiss and Shrout, 1977) and found: $R_A = 0.97$, $R_B = 0.83$, $R_C = 0.84$. When the R values were computed separately on the basis of the data from the group of patients and the group of staff members, the R values were somewhat reduced, but were still sufficiently high (Sundsvold et al, 1982).

The reliability of the sum scores of the 12 categories was also computed. The results of the 12 categories are shown in Table 2.1, where the inter-tester reliability between physical therapist A and B, and A and C is computed by help of the RHO coefficient. The results both from the 12 categories and the single examinations show the highest concensus between the physical therapist A and B about ranking of the person's muscle status on the basis of the sum score of each category. As expected, the concensus is highest between physical therapist A and B. Stretch palpation was the category that gave the lowest RHO score between A and B. We have therefore somewhat changed the technique of stretch palpation to make it easier to learn and to raise the reliability.

Table 2.1 Intertester reliability of the sum scores of the GPM categories of muscle examinations. RHO-coefficient between physical therapists A and B and between A and C.

Methods	Categories	A and B	A and C
Posture	Standing	0.75	0.79
	Supine position	0.66	0.53
	Passive range of movements	0.71	0.35
Respiration	Amplitude of inspiration	0.71	0.35
Movements	Passive movements against gravity with active stimulus by therapist	0.86	0.83
	Passive movements	0.84	0.68
	Active range of movements	0.78	0.72
Palpation	Stretch palpation	0.50	0.47
	Pressure palpation	0.89	0.46
	Subjective reaction to stretch palpation	0.75	0.77

So far the findings from this study have shown that it is possible for physical therapists to learn the GPM method and thereby to rank the same persons in the same way. Examining the raw scores showed, however, that physical therapist C (with the least experience) used the scale in a somewhat different way than the others. She did not use the extremes of the scales as much as the physical therapists A and B. The mean of her total sum scores was 1.89 (SD =

0.75) while the mean of A's was 2.87 (SD = 0.9) and B's 2.62 (SD = 0.80). These findings show that the two most experienced physical therapists also used the scales most similarily. It demonstrates the necessity of systematic training and supervision to learn the GPM method. It also shows that if one wants to compare the findings in different patients or combine the findings of two or more physical therapists in one study, it is important to be sure that the scales are used in the same way.

DEVIANT MUSCLE CONDITIONS AND ASSESSMENT OF PSYCHOPATHOLOGY

Using the GPM method, a study has been made of the relationship between deviant muscle conditions and psychopathology in four separate research projects. The studies include 445 persons of both sexes, divided into four groups with different degrees of psychopathology: psychotic inpatients, neurotic and borderline inpatients, out-patients seen at a physical therapy private office and healthy control groups. These projects are described and most of the results are reported in a recent paper (Sundsvold & Vaglum, 1982) which also contains an extensive description of our earlier research. We will here only give a summary of the findings:

1. A systematic relationship was found between the frequency of deviant muscle findings and the degree of psychopathology. The psychotic inpatients had the highest frequency of deviant muscle findings, next came the borderline and the ego-weak neurotic inpatients, then came the group of out-patients from a private physical therapy office, and the lowest frequency of deviant findings was found in the healthy control groups. As to the frequency of painful reactions to stretch palpation, we found the same pattern of results.

2. In the group of hospitalized psychiatric inpatients, the sum score of the category examining movements, discriminated significantly between psychotic patients and neurotic patients (Sundsvold et al, 1981). A differention between psychotic and neurotic patients was also possible based on the results of the assessment of respiration (Sundsvold et al, 1980).

3. Among the hospitalized non-psychotic patients, those with a borderline diagnosis (Gunderson and Singer, 1975) reported more indifferent reactions than the ego-weak neurotics when they were stretch palpated (Sundsvold & Vaglum, 1982).

4. In the group of hospitalized non-psychotic patients, the lower

the score for deviant muscle findings on admission, the more likely it was that the patient was discharged as he improved. In a group of female drug abusers, there was also a significant relationship between the muscle conditions on admission and the degree of drug abuse 3–5 years after discharge. The less deviant muscle findings the patient had on admission to the hospital, the lower the drug abuse was 3–5 years after discharge.

The research in this field is only in its beginning stages. The studies show, however, that the GPM examination gives information about more than the muscle and somatic status. The total sum score of the patient may also be used for assessing the degree of psychopathology. The exact size of the total sum score that should be considered as a definite sign of a high degree of psychopathology, or should be considered as a warning signal for a threatening psychological break-down, is, however, not yet possible to define exactly. More research is needed. Some of our findings up to now may, however, give us some help:

Figure 2.2 indicates the distribution of the total sum score of the GPM in four groups of people which are known to have a different degree of psychopathology. The solid lines indicate the area covering approximately 68% of the persons of the group (±1 SD). The dotted lines indicate the full range of the findings in the group. Each group consists of 30 people, and the distribution of men and women is approximately 33% men and 66% women. The group of young schizophrenic inpatients consists of mostly subchronic schizophrenic inpatients, all of them inpatients in a mental hospital. The neurotic and borderline patients of the day hospital are a group exhibiting some ego-weakness, but the degree of psychopathology is less than in the schizophrenic group. The patients from the physical therapy practice are mainly ego-strong neurotic patients, while only 10% of the group of the control persons had a moderate degree of neurotic problems. The means and the range of the total sum scores of the four groups are seen in Table 2.2.

The findings presented in Table 2.2 and Figure 2.2 show that the higher the group's degree of psychopathology is, the more deviant are the muscle findings. It shows, however, also that there is a great overlap as to the distribution of the sum scores of the different groups. This indicates that it is not possible to use the total sum score of a certain patient to make a specific psychiatric diagnosis. The GPM total sum score is only indicating the degree of psychopathology of a person, not the type. Within a psychiatric diagnostic group which indicates both the degree and type of psychopathol-

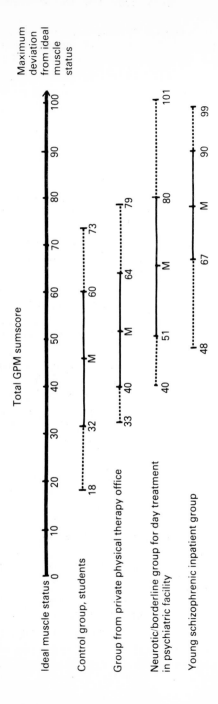

Fig. 2.2 The Global Physiotherapeutic muscle examination's assessment scale for the degree of psychopathology. The distribution of GPM's total sumscore in four groups with different degree of psychopathology. (range, M = mean). The area of ± 1 SD

Table 2.2 The results from the GPM total sum score showing the mean (M), the standard deviation (SD), limit of ± 1 SD*, sum score range and age range.

Group N = 30	M	SD	Limit of ± 1 SD*	Sum score range
Control group, students (functionally healthy)	46	14	32–60	18–73
Patients seen in private practice, physical therapy office	52	12	40–64	33–79
Neurotic/borderline patients coming for day treatment in psychiatric facility	65	14	51–80	40–101
Young schizophrenic inpatients	78	11	67–90	48–99

* ± 1 SD = approximately 68% of the group

ogy, the GPM may, however, discriminate between patients with different degrees of psychopathology. Some of our earlier studies have shown that those patients within a certain psychiatric diagnostic group which have the less deviant muscle findings on admission, also had a tendency to have a better outcome at discharge and at follow-up. The GPM total sum score may, therefore, give valuable information which is supplemental to the psychiatric diagnosis. More research is needed.

The results in Figure 2.2 show also the fact that some few patients with a psychiatric diagnosis which indicates a high degree of psychopathology, may have a relatively low GPM total sum score (between 40 and 55). This means that one cannot exclude a serious psychiatric condition only on the basis of the GPM total sum score. In a physical therapy private practice, such psychiatric patients with low sum scores can be identified only by soliciting more data in the interview. On the other hand, if the GPM total sum score is more than 55 in non-psychiatric patients, experience has shown that such patients usually have greater psychological problems than they are able to cope with. The higher the total sum score is, the higher may the patient's degree of psychopathology be. The GPM total sum score may disclose a present or earlier psychiatric condition which the patient has forgotten, avoids talking about, or has never sought help for previously. This shows again the importance of also doing extensive examinations of the patient's social functioning, life situation and mental health, before treatment planning.

Before describing the evaluation of two patients as an example of the use of the GPM muscle examination, a brief discussion will be presented on the importance of the case history as one of the bases of evaluation and treatment planning.

THE CASE HISTORY

Taking a good and relevant case history is a part of the art of physical therapy. We can here only underline some of the important points which are related to the evaluation of patients with muscular pains. The aim of the interview is to establish a good patient–therapist relationship, and collect detailed information about the development and localization of the muscular pains, and information relevant for diagnosing neurological diseases and diseases of the joints. The interview should give the physical therapist a picture of the present and former social functioning and mental health of the patient. The therapist should look for a relationship between stressful life events and the precipitation of muscular pains and somatic and psychological symptoms, both in the past and in the present situation. To get an overview of possible relationships between life events, mental health problems and muscular pains (and other somatic disorders), it is useful to record the information in the type of diagram which is shown for case II in Figure 2.6. On the left side of the vertical life axis are presented the somatic or psychological symptoms at different points in time. On the right side of the vertical life axis are the points in time of important life events and alterations in social functioning. As an example the reader may see that case II (Fig. 2.6) has a tendency to get muscular pains and symptoms every time she gets into situations where she gets more personal obligations.

SELECTION OF TREATMENT

In addition to the GPM results, the disclosure of a relationship between stressful life situations and muscular pains and other symptoms, also gives the physical therapist important information needed for treatment planning. The following are two examples.

1. If the patient is in a conflicting life situation which cannot be altered in the near future, it may make the situation even worse for the patient if the physical therapist tries to eliminate the local muscular pain without helping the patient to cope with the situation psychologically as well as somatically. Before the selection of treatment methods, the physical therapist, therefore, must evaluate how much the patient needs the tightened, painful muscles as a part of her/his defense mechanism. On the basis of our studies and clinical experience, it is recommended that active movements be used and not relaxation therapy if the patient has a total sum score higher

than 55. If the sum score is below 55, it is still recommended that the same type of treatment be used if the patient is in a stressful life situation and/or exhibits reduced social functioning and/or psychiatric symptoms. If passive relaxation therapy is given in both cases, it is necessary that the physical therapist collaborates with a psychiatrist or a psychotherapist (Houge, 1978).

2. Some patients may on earlier occasions have had one or more nervous breakdowns. The physical therapist in such cases should start the therapy with active methods. Even if patients are treated with active movements without intention of relaxation, the treatment may still cause a relaxation response. In this case, the patient himself generally is more able to control the degree of relaxation he can tolerate, and he will usually not relax more than he can bear. The physical therapist still has to be careful with the dosage of the treatment.

The active methods recommended in these cases are often supportive of the postural muscles, helping the patient to 'stand on his feet'. Physical therapy is by no means contraindicated by manifest psychiatric disorders such as neurosis, borderline-states, substance abuse or psychosis. In such cases, it is, however, especially important to consider the total muscular condition, and to use active treatment methods which both strengthen and limber the muscles without dissolving the muscular defenses. The following are two case histories taken from private physical therapy practice. The cases exemplify the use of the GPM examination in evaluation and treatment planning. The first patient has clearly more deviant muscle findings than the second one.

CASE 1

A WOMAN WITH LOW BACK PAIN

GPM evaluation

Mrs A, a 35-year-old married woman, was referred by a general practitioner (GP) to a private physical therapy office for relaxation treatment because of low back pain. She had experienced low back pain intermittently during the past 2 years. Except for these pains, she had never been to see a doctor. The pains were located primarily in the lumbosacral region, but sometimes also in the lower part of the thoracic column. During the last months, the pains were constantly present during the day, being somewhat stronger in the late evenings and the mornings. For the last four weeks she had had to stay at home, unable to do her job as a private secretary.

Results of the single examination in the GPM

Inspection of posture

In the standing position, the lumbar lordosis L1–5 was a little too curved and the thoracal kyphosis Th9–12 was too flat. The waist and the lateral epigastric region were very tight. In the supine position the lumbar lordosis was totally straightened out. Maximal passive flexion of the hip joints was 78° and did not cause pain. A sciatic disorder could be excluded.

Inspection of respiration

In standing position the amplitude of inspiration in the hypogastric, the lateral epigastric and the lower lateral costal regions was not visible. A small inspirational amplitude was observed in the medial epigastric region. In the high costal region the amplitude was too extended. The rhythm was rough and the frequency was too fast. In supine the inspirational amplitude was only a little inhibited in all five regions. Rhythm and frequency were good.

Examination of movements

With her m.gluteus maximus towards the wall, standing idle with trunk and head bent forwards and knee stretched, passive gravity movements of head/cervical and lumbosacral regions were extremely inhibited. She had very little ability to let herself relax or release in these regions in response to manual pressure from the therapist. Passive leading movements of lower and upper extremities were also inhibited. She had little ability to let herself be led through a movement by the therapist. The maximal extent of active range of movement in the feet were highly restricted. Only the maximal extent of active range of movement of the jaw was adequate.

Evaluation by palpation

Findings from stretch palpation showed muscles which were too short and tightened, in m.gastrocnemius, the radialis group, m.pectoralis lateralis, the teres group and m.sacrospinalis C3–5. Sacrospinalis L2–4 was only a little too short and tightened. Stretch palpation caused much pain and discomfort in all palpated muscles. Press palpation showed deviations in a negative direction in all the muscles, i.e. the muscles felt as if they were too 'dry'. The skin was also a little too dry. The single examinations in all categories showed that the deviations were not only present in the back where she had her pains, but were distributed throughout the entire body. During the examination the physical therapist observed that the patient was talking with a low voice and answering questions very slowly.

Sum scores of the 12 categories

The sum scores of the 12 categories of this patient are shown in Figure 2.3. We can see that the patient shows most deviations in 3 categories: too many painful reactions to stretch palpations, too great an inhibition of movements and too great an inhibition of respiration in the standing position. Many painful reactions to stretch palpation indicate that she might be in a stressful life situation. Deviations in movements and respiration have also been shown in our clinical research to discriminate fairly well between patients with different degrees of psychopathology. The inhibition of the respiration and the distribution of deviant findings, may also indicate that she tries to control her feelings.

Total sum score

The total sum score of this patient is 64. Looking at the scale in Figure 2.2 we see that the total sum score of this patient, 64, lies at the upper limit of approximately 68% of the group of patients seen in a private physical therapy office, near the mean in a group of psychiatric day inpatients and near the lower limit of approximately 68% of the schizophrenic group of inpatients. This indicates that the patient may have a mental disorder, and a thorough exploration of the patient's life situation, social functioning and mental health became very important prior to treatment planning and actual therapy.

Case history

In the interview the patient told us that she had been somewhat anxious since childhood with an exaggeration of symptoms during

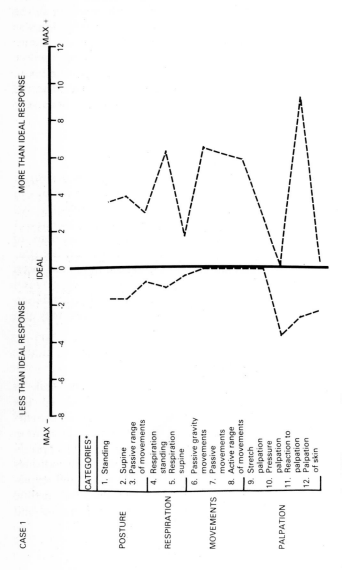

Fig. 2.3 The sumscores of 12 categories in the GPM-examination showing the muscle pattern of a patient with low back pain.

her pregnancy 10 years ago. (For more details see Fig. 2.4.) She had always felt a bit inferior intellectually, and got low marks in high-school. At 18 years of age she married a man who over the years established a very good career in the military service which entailed moving house frequently. The husband was very occupied with his job. Three years ago she took a secretarial training course and got a well-paid job as a secretary. Soon after beginning her job she fell in love with one of the directors and had an affair with him. She felt constantly guilty and anxious that her husband should discover this affair, and for the last 6 months she had wanted to stop the affair without managing to do so.

Treatment

The information gathered in the interview confirmed GPM findings that the patient was in a very conflicting life situation where she possibly needed her muscular inhibitions (armour) to manage the situation. The low back pain might also be seen as a way of coping with the situation: the pain made her stay away from the job and her lover. The physician had ordered relaxation therapy. Because of her actual stressful life situation, her relatively high total sum score, 64, her high frequency of muscles with palpational pains distributed throughout the entire body, and her inhibited movements and respiration, it was contraindicated to start with a general or localized relaxation therapy. Instead, she was given a treatment program consisting of active movements of the lower extremities where the main point was to limber her stiff feet. She was also given walking exercises with her attention focused on how she used and felt her feet and legs during walking and in the standing position. She had to learn 'to stay on her feet'. In addition, she got some rapid swing exercises for the upper extremities and some rapid stimulating massage of her legs. The feet, especially, were worked on. She was encouraged to be acquainted with her body and how it reacted during the exercises and to talk about it. If the patient asked for advice other than about exercises, she was never advised on what to do, she had to find out herself. The dosage of the treatment was evaluated continuously during the whole therapy. She was told to stop the exercises if she felt uncomfortable. She also exercised at home. The first two weeks she was treated twice a week, later only once. This type of physical therapy usually loosens up the muscle armour very slowly, and not faster than the patient can tolerate. The patient has the control herself. After one month

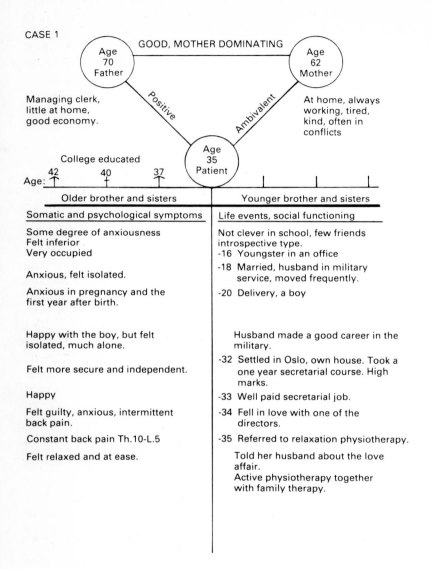

CASE 1

GOOD, MOTHER DOMINATING

Age 70 Father — Age 62 Mother

Managing clerk, little at home, good economy.

Positive   *Ambivalent*

At home, always working, tired, kind, often in conflicts

Age 35 Patient

College educated

Age: 42 40 37

Older brother and sisters | Younger brother and sisters

Somatic and psychological symptoms	Life events, social functioning
Some degree of anxiousness Felt inferior Very occupied	Not clever in school, few friends introspective type. -16 Youngster in an office
Anxious, felt isolated.	-18 Married, husband in military service, moved frequently.
Anxious in pregnancy and the first year after birth.	-20 Delivery, a boy
Happy with the boy, but felt isolated, much alone.	Husband made a good career in the military.
Felt more secure and independent.	-32 Settled in Oslo, own house. Took a one year secretarial course. High marks.
Happy	-33 Well paid secretarial job.
Felt guilty, anxious, intermittent back pain.	-34 Fell in love with one of the directors.
Constant back pain Th.10-L.5	-35 Referred to relaxation physiotherapy.
Felt relaxed and at ease.	Told her husband about the love affair. Active physiotherapy together with family therapy.

Fig. 2.4 Case history describing somatic and psychological symptoms, life events and social functioning of a patient with low back pain.

of physical therapy she broke up with her lover, and told her husband about the love affair. They decided to go to family therapy in parallel with physical therapy. After some family therapy sessions the active methods and rapid massage was given more distinctly for the trunk and upper extremity, and lastly the neck and head were incorporated in the treatment.

CASE 2

A WOMAN WITH PAIN IN THE CHEST

A 59-year-old married housewife was referred from a physician to physical therapy for respiration exercises because of persisting pain in the left side of the chest. Cardiac diseases had been excluded. The pains were present throughout the day, and had been slowly worsening during the last year. She had experienced such pains twice earlier in her life, at the age of 22 and 30.

Results of the single examinations by GPM

Inspection of posture

In standing position the waist and the lateral epigastrium were drawn in. The high costal thorax had little extension. In supine the medial low costal thoracic region showed little extension and the flexion of the shoulders was a little too great.

Inspection of respiration

The inspirational amplitude in standing position was fairly visible in the medial hypogastric and lateral epigastric regions, while the high costal amplitude was too great. In lying supine the respiration was adequate.

Examinations of movements

There were only small deviations. Only the feet were a little too stiff.

Evaluation by palpation

Stretch palpation showed too short and tightened muscles in m.triceps, m.sacrospinalis, Th10–12. The rest of the muscles were adequate in response to stretching of muscles. However, stretch palpation released pains in the entire body. The circulation in muscles and skin was only a little too dry. Most deviations in all categories were found in the thorax/upper extremity region of this patient. During the examination the physical therapist got the impression of an open, warm and responsible woman.

Sum scores of the 12 categories

The results from the 12 assessment categories is shown in Figure 2.5. There are only moderate deviations in the findings of all the 12 categories. Only the subjective pains released by stretch palpation were too high. Passive movements and posture were most nearly adequate.

Total sum score

The total sum score was 43, placing this patient just within the lower limit of approximately 68% of the group of patients at the private physical therapy office. The muscular findings indicate that this might be a patient with a relatively small degree of psychopathology. But her relatively high frequency of palpational painful muscles indicate that she may be in a stressful situation.

Case history

The patient had had an ambivalent relationship with her mother since childhood. The chest pains had started when her elderly mother had a stroke and became so helpless that the patient had to take her into her own house and care for her constantly for half a year. It was now nearly one year since her mother died, but the pains were unchanged. The patient had always been somewhat anxious, especially if she got new obligations. She had, however, never contacted a doctor for her anxiety, and neither had she used any medication. Her first incident of chest pains occurred the first half-year after she had her child. The second occurred the first half-year after her husband was appointed as managing director of a big firm. Her relationship with her husband and children was happy and uncomplicated. She said that she felt relieved when her mother died. (For more details see Fig. 2.6.)

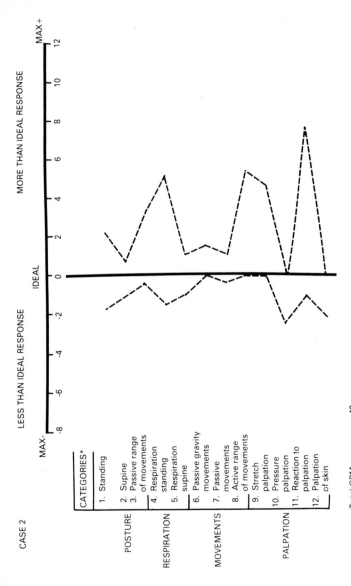

Fig. 2.5 The sumscores of 12 categories in the GPM-examination showing the muscle pattern of a patient with chest pain.

CASE 2

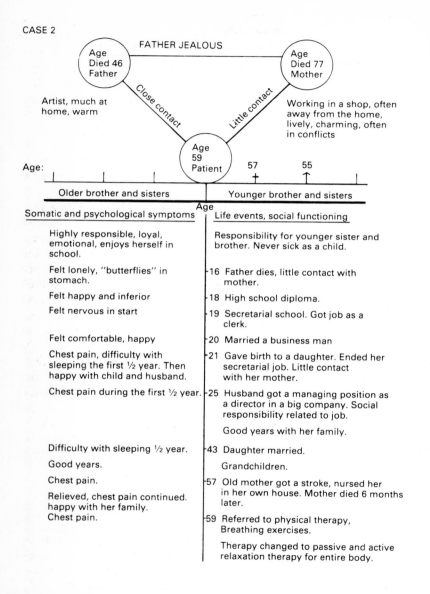

Somatic and psychological symptoms	Life events, social functioning
Highly responsible, loyal, emotional, enjoys herself in school.	Responsibility for younger sister and brother. Never sick as a child.
Felt lonely, "butterflies" in stomach.	16 Father dies, little contact with mother.
Felt happy and inferior	18 High school diploma.
Felt nervous in start	19 Secretarial school. Got job as a clerk.
Felt comfortable, happy	20 Married a business man
Chest pain, difficulty with sleeping the first ½ year. Then happy with child and husband.	21 Gave birth to a daughter. Ended her secretarial job. Little contact with her mother.
Chest pain during the first ½ year.	25 Husband got a managing position as a director in a big company. Social responsibility related to job.
	Good years with her family.
Difficulty with sleeping ½ year.	43 Daughter married.
Good years.	Grandchildren.
Chest pain.	57 Old mother got a stroke, nursed her in her own house. Mother died 6 months later.
Relieved, chest pain continued. happy with her family. Chest pain.	59 Referred to physical therapy, Breathing exercises.
	Therapy changed to passive and active relaxation therapy for entire body.

Fig. 2.6 Case history describing somatic and psychological symptoms, life events and social functioning of a patient with chest pain.

Treatment

The GPM findings and the case history showed that this was a woman with many resources both in her muscles and psychologically. Her present life situation seemed to be uncomplicated. Her chest pains seemed to be precipitated in situations when she got new obligations. Her latent anxiety then became mobilized. The last time this was precipitated was by her mother's sickness and her need for care. The muscles of respiration were obviously used to control this anxiety. At present she did not experience her life situation as stressful, and did not feel any anxiety. Her chest muscles were, however, still very tight as if she still was in an anxiety-provoking situation. This phenomenon may be seen as a muscular wedlock phenomenon. The stress situation was over, but muscular pains continued because her muscular armour was not able to relax.

Both the GPM and the case history and social functioning showed that this patient had many resources, and should be able to tolerate both a passive and active relaxation therapy. The main aim of the physical therapy was to loosen up her muscles in the thoracic/upper extremity regions and let her feel and learn how to relax. Instead of giving her breathing exercises the therapy was changed to relaxation therapy of the entire body one hour a week. The treatment consisted of soft slow massage all over the body in parallel with the respiration, broken up with passive movements and vibration. In the standing position in front of a mirror her attention was called to her constantly tightened abdomen. She was told how much this led to restriction of her respiration, and the connection between this restraint and her chest pains. She was trained to 'let her stomach go', and given stretching exercises in parallel with audible sighs. At last she was taught the general relaxation therapy ad modum Dick-Read (1960) in the breathing rhythm with audible sighs, and she was told to practice at home.

CONCLUSION

Painful muscles and localized pains on palpation may be found in patients with both minor and major emotional disorders. The localized muscle tenderness/pains found on palpation of the muscle are usually not pains which the patient will feel during normal daily activity, and are therefore not usually reported as a problem by the patient. Patients complaining of localized muscular pain frequently on examination have pains on palpation in other parts of the body.

Also, a high frequency of localized pain on palpation may indicate that the patient's life situation is difficult to cope with. A high frequency of indifferent or neutral reactions to stretch palpation may on the other hand indicate that the patient has poor contact with his own body and his own feelings. The patient's complaints of localized muscle pains may be a symptom of a general pattern of muscle deviations. It is therefore important to make an evaluation of the muscle status throughout the entire body before a decision is made as to the type of therapeutic intervention.

The GPM method gives both a systematic description of muscle status throughout the entire body and an indication of the degree of psychopathology based on a numerical rating scale of muscle status. The higher the total GPM sum score is, the more variation from ideal muscle status and the higher the degree of psychopathology may be. If the total GPM sum score is higher than 55, the patient's muscle status is dysfunctional, and clinical experiences have shown that he usually also has more emotional problems than he manages to cope with.

When the total GPM sum score is higher than 55, caution must be exercized as to the type of physical therapy used in order to avoid creating more emotional strain on the patient, and/or avoid contributing to a nervous breakdown. Physical therapists should always be careful with the use of relaxation therapy. If the total sum score is higher than 55, if the patient is in an acute stressful life situation and if the patient has had a nervous breakdown, active methods should be used initially. Combined with a case history describing somatic and psychological symptoms, life events and social functioning, GPM can provide a sound basis for planning therapeutic interventions.

There is still much research to be done before we know enough about the relationship between muscular pains, muscular status and mental health, and about which patients with which muscular conditions should have which type of therapeutic intervention. It is our experience that the GPM method is a valuable tool in clinical practice as well as in clinical research for the study of stress-related diseases, sports medicine, postural deviations in children and adults, and the outcome of different types of physical therapy.

REFERENCES

Aiken P A 1980 Muscle and personality I: properties of muscle. The Journal of Biological Experience 2: 41–55

Basmajian J V Muscles alive: their functions revealed by electromyography, 4th edn. Williams and Wilkins, Baltimore

Braatøy T 1954 Fundamentals of psychoanalytic technique. Wiley, New York

Bülow Hansen A 1967 Problemer ved behandling av muskel-spenninger. Norsk Tannlægeforenings Tidsskrift 1: 6–13

Dick-Read G 1960 Childbirth without fear. William Heinemann Medical Books Ltd, London

Fleiss J L, Shrout P E 1977 The effects of measurement errors on some multivariate procedures. American Journal of Public Health 67: 1188–1191

Gunderson J G, Singer M S 1975 Defining borderline patients: an overview. American Journal of psychiatry 132: 1–10

Houge N 1978 Physiotherapy in certain aspects of psychosomatic medicine. Paper at the XIIth European Conference on Psychosomatic Research, Bodø, Sweden

Karterud S 1980 Følelsesmessige reaksjoner ved fysikalsk behandling. En pilotstudie. Tidsskrift for Den Norske Lægeforening 100: 220–223

Lowen A 1958 Physical dynamics of character structure. Greene and Stratton, New York.

Reich W 1950 Character analysis. Farrer, Strauss, Gironx, New York.

Sundsvold M 1969 Muskelundersøkelse ved psykiske sykdommer. Fysioterapeuten 36: 68–79.

Sundsvold M 1975 Muscular tension and psychopathology. Psychotherapy and Psychosomatics 26: 219–228.

Sundsvold M 1976 Muskelpalpasjon som undersøkelsesmetode. Fysioterapeuten 43: 383–388.

Sundsvold M Ø, Vaglum P, Ostberg B 1976 Clinical muscle characteristics and psychopathology. I. A comparison between four groups of person with a different type and degree of psychopathology. Paper presented at the 11th European Conference on Psychosomatic Research, Heidelberg.

Sundsvold M Ø, Vaglum P, Østberg B 1980 Respirasjon og psykopatologi. Fysioterapeuten 47: 103–107.

Sundsvold M Ø, Vaglum P, Østberg B 1981 Movements, lumbar and temporomandibular pains and psychopathology. Psychotherapy and Psychosomatics 35: 1–8.

Sundsvold M Ø, Vaglum P, Denstad K 1982 Global Fysioterapeutisk Muskelundersøkelse. Til bruk i klinisk arbeid og forskning. Eget forlag, Oslo, pp. 211.

Sundsvold M Ø, Vaglum P, 1982 Muscle characteristics and psychopathology: II. Three studies of psychotic, ego-weak neurotic and abusing patients using the GPM examination. Proceedings The IXth International Congress of World Confederation for Physical Therapy, Stockholm, pp 221–226.

Psychological approaches to the treatment of chronic pain

> Pain is not a simple affair of an impulse travelling at a fixed rate along a nerve. It is the resultant of a conflict between a stimulus and the whole individual.
>
> Leriche, surgeon, late 19th century.

PHILOSOPHY OF PAIN

The word 'pain' is difficult to define. The medical meaning, to which physiotherapists adhere, is that pain is organic, but if this is so, why is there 'no simple direct relationship between the wound *per se* and the pain experienced'? (Beecher, 1966)

Pain can be described as a sensation of a special sort that we ordinarily dislike (see Ryle, 1949). A person learns about pain through experience, and whatever he feels on those occasions when he naturally manifests pain he is taught to call *pain*. Since the child learns the word *pain* on occasions when he feels something that he wants to stop or reduce in intensity, or of whose return he is afraid, the meaning of the word *pain* becomes 'something which I dislike'. Because pain is almost universally disliked and because this fact is depended upon in order to reach the concept, the word *pain* can be used to refer to the total experience of both sensation and emotion (see Baier, in Trigg, 1970).

Melzack (1973), who developed the Gate Control Theory of Pain, said that to consider pain only as a sensation was a relatively recent occurrence and that the older theory, dating back to Aristotle, considered pain to be an emotion—the opposite of pleasure—rather than a sensation. He noted that pain was not just a sensory quality but also had a strong negative affective quality that drove the subject into activity. However, the remarkable development of sensory physiology and psychophysics and of technical equipment like X-ray machines and scanners during the 20th century has given momentum to the concept of pain as a sensation and has overshadowed the role of affective and motivational processes. Nevertheless, the sensory approach to pain, valuable as it may have been, has failed to provide a complete picture of pain processes: the assumption that pain was primarily a sensation relegated motivational and cognitive processes to the role of *reaction to pain* and made them only *secondary considerations* to the whole pain process. Melzack concluded that sensory, motivational and cognitive processes occurred concurrently in parallel, interacting systems and that motivational/affective processes must be included in any satisfactory theory of pain. A treatment plan, therefore, must include concurrent interventions for organic, emotional and behavioural aspects of pain.

Three levels of pain are given by Szasz (1968) in his model. One is a biological level in which the concept of pain is that of a signal by which the perceptual part of the organism registers that there is a threat to its structural and functional integrity: in this concept of pain there is only one person involved. Two or more people are involved at another level in which the expression of pain is a fundamental method of asking for help. In the third aspect, the meaning of the word *pain* lies largely in its communicative aspect. Pain, in this context, may not denote a reference to the body; it may then function as affect or emotion.

The pairing of the words *pain* and *suffering* is discussed by Cassell (1982) who says that this phenomenon reflects a historically constrained and currently inadequate view of the ends of medicine. Medicine's traditional primary concern for the body and for physical disease is well known, as are the widespread effects of the mind-body dichotomy on medical theory and practice. Medicine has relegated pain to the body and suffering to the mind, and today, as ideals of the separation of mind and body are called into question, physicians are concerning themselves with new aspects of the human condition. Cassell says that suffering is experienced by persons and that the understanding of the person in human illness requires a rejection of the historic dualism of mind and body. The *person* in pain frequently reports suffering from pain when he feels out of control, when the source of the pain is unknown, when the meaning of the pain is dire or when the pain is chronic. In all these situations subjects perceive pain as a threat to their continued existence—not merely to their lives but to their integrity as persons. Cassell concludes that this relation of pain to suffering must be acknowledged because suffering can be relieved, in the presence of continual pain, by making the source of the pain known, by

changing its meaning and by demonstrating that it can be controlled and that an end is in sight.

Physiotherapists, when challenged by chronic pain, must also
relieve suffering by treating the whole person. Treatment of a
specific part of the body alone will not suffice.

TREATMENT MODEL

The primary aim of treatment is to prevent chronic pain from becoming a chronic disability; alleviation of the pain is a secondary
aim.

Pain, whatever its cause, is a source of stress; it is associated with
irritability and anxiety (Moon, 1981a) which is shown in body posture; the body tends to flex with shoulders elevated, limbs ad-
ducted, jaw clenched, forehead wrinkled and breathing controlled.
This posturing over long periods results in muscle fatigue with increased discomfort, especially if superimposed on the pain site; and
so the pain increases. Thus, a simple loop is formed; pain induces
stress, the expression of which perpetuates the pain.

Other events in the subject's life may also be causing stress and
it is important to note that the word *stress* is not necessarily *dis-
stress*; happy events like a wedding or a job promotion also cause
stress. Stress is not necessarily dramatic but is a function of everyday life and relates to stimulation and challenge, without which life
would be lifeless! A simple explanation of the nature of stress must
be given to the patient (see Cox, 1978; Selye, 1975).

The pain causes the subject to hold the body awkwardly or stiffly
as a protection against knocks that could increase the pain. Postural
habits develop that give muscle imbalances that increase the disability caused by the pain. Unnecessary exercise will be avoided,
with a loss of physical fitness and a decrease in the sense of
wellbeing.

These changes effect performance both at work and within the
family with a lowering of self-esteem and distress; another loop in
the pain-pattern forms.

Therefore, in assessing the patient who presents for treatment of
chronic pain, it is the pain-pattern concerning the whole person
within his environment, rather than a specific pain, that must be
noted (Fig. 3.1). The essential components of the pain-pattern are
the pain site itself, the emotion that is inherent in that pain and the
body behaviour that expresses that emotion in a manner that perpetuates the pain. The patient must grasp the concept of pain-

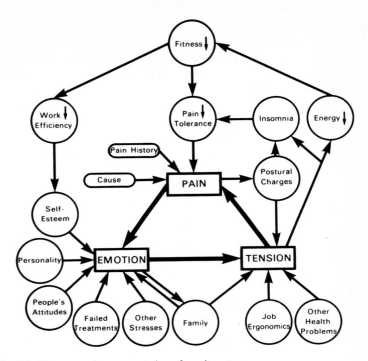

Fig. 3.1 Diagrammatic representation of a pain-pattern.

pattern in order to be able to accept that treatment will be aimed at altering this pain-pattern rather than at curing the specific pain.

To summarise so far, the treatment model for chronic pain entails a *pain-pattern* rather than a *pain*. The principal component of this pain-pattern is the simple loop in which pain causes stress that is expressed in the muscle system in a manner which perpetuates the pain. Other current life events causing stress can activate this loop. Postural habits develop that decrease the efficiency of the body and can lead to a decline in the ability to function in the job and family. Stress increases; so does the pain.

Once the concept of the pain-pattern is accepted the patient has to understand his role in treatment. Classically, when pain is considered to be organic the patient is relegated to a passive role to be the recipient of treatment given by experts who are trained to examine, understand and heal the body. Indeed, this role is inherent in the derivation of the word *patient*, which comes from the Latin word 'to suffer'. *Patience* means *inter alia*, 'calm endurance of pain or any provocation' (Concise Oxford Dictionary). As diligent involvement is required if a person is to alter his pain-pattern the word *patient* is inappropriate; the person with chronic pain works in a partnership with the therapist; that person must become motivated to take full responsibility for his pain and to participate actively in the program in order to ensure a positive outcome. In this article, henceforth, the word patient will be used only in patient-situations.

Treatment goals must be realistic. Usually, a person with chronic pain has seen many therapists from various disciplines and is waiting for a cure. In the early stages of treatment, confrontation is often necessary. Thus the therapist may say that the pain will not be taken away, but that skills will be taught to permit more effective handling of the pain situation. Thus, a lesser goal is set: one that has some chance of being attained. Any small sense of achievement so gained gives confidence, ensures continuing participation and decreases anxiety, thereby initiating changes in the pain-pattern.

Thus, the concept of *pain-pattern* is to be preferred rather than *pain*. The person with pain is a *partner* in treatment rather than a *patient*. The initial goal is to improve the skill of *handling* pain rather than to cure pain.

LITERATURE REVIEW

Leavitt (1978) used Melzack and Torgeson's (1971) adjective list in a study of chronic back pain to show the inclusion of *emotion* in the meaning of the word *pain*. Acute pain, after hysterectomy, was studied similarly. (Moon, 1982a).

Pain was viewed as learned behaviour by Fordyce (1973) in a study of chronic pain in which he looked for reinforcers for pain behaviour. He considered that the diagnostic process should examine the relationships between pain behaviour and both pathogenic factors and systematic environmental consequences.

Muscle behaviour expresses emotion. Mitchell (1977) described the posture of the body in fear while Schwartz and Fair (1976) showed how facial muscle action differentiated happiness and sadness.

The use of relaxation training to reduce anxiety is based on Wolpe's (1958) theory of psychotherapy by reciprocal inhibition in which he said anxiety and relaxation were antagonistic entities. Smith (1973) showed a positive correlation between trait anxiety and EMG measured by electrodes placed on the frontalis muscle.

Moon (1982a) showed that forehead muscle activity reflected levels of trait anxiety and also that relaxation behaviour was antagonistic to irritability.

Various studies have examined the use of relaxation training (Grzesiak, 1977) and of EMG biofeedback-mediated relaxation training (Wickramasekera, 1972; Hendler, 1977) in the treatment of chronic pain. Turk (1979) reviewed studies of pain and biofeedback training and said that biofeedback was rarely used alone and he noted the importance of home practice.

EMG biofeedback as a method used to train people to alter muscle patterns of activity was seen by Arbogast (1978) to have possibly its greatest advantage in its diagnostic function. Traditional psychotherapy may take many hours to establish a link between some emotional stress and a physiological event whereas, with biofeedback techniques, that link between mind and body can be more rapidly detected.

Older (1983) wrote that he was one who believed that the mind-body split which assigns psychiatrists to the psyche and physiotherapists to the soma was artificial and undesirable. Worse still, by making body contact taboo to the psychiatrist and psychological exploration equally taboo to the physiotherapist, holistic care (in the best sense of the phrase) was rendered impossible.

TREATMENT PLAN

Referral

Patients should be referred after a thorough physical assessment, preferably by a physician, to ascertain the presence or nature of organic components of the pain.

Length of treatment sessions

Time is required to listen to the patient, to assess all aspects of the pain-pattern and to initiate a multiple-treatment plan. Therefore, individual treatment sessions of 50–60 minutes are necessary.

Frequency of treatment sessions

Assessment of complex problems along with the establishment of trust may require two treatment sessions a week for the first week or so. Usually, treatment once a week is sufficient as responsibility for carrying out treatment rests with the person with pain and not with the physiotherapist. After 3–4 weeks, if there is a positive response, occasional follow-up sessions usually are all that are required.

Duration of treatment

Duration depends on the complexity of the problem, but with an active partnership between the person with pain and the therapist, about 3–4 sessions will initiate changes, and a further 1–2 follow-up sessions will ensure the continuation of these changes. It is important to avoid the development of a dependent situation because the treatment partnership would thereby give way to the therapist-patient relationship.

Termination of treatment

Once positive changes are occurring, discharge will be by common agreement between the two parties. There is no need to keep treatment going until complete relief of pain is obtained.

When a patient is unmotivated and takes no responsibility, he will usually break the treatment contract after one or two sessions anyway. Some people are either unwilling or unable or not ready to take responsibility. Other supportive treatment may be more applicable.

If a person attends with no changes or a deterioration of pain behaviour then, providing a full physical assessment has already been made, it may be appropriate to refer that patient for a psychological assessment.

If a person is attending regularly and appears to be participating but the therapist is not sure whether progress is being made, then two strategies can be used. A contract of, say, another three appointments can be given, which may increase motivation. Alternatively, instead of scheduling further appointments, the person with pain can be asked to telephone for an occasional appointment if required. These follow-up appointments may be to re-assess the treatment situation or to give support and encouragement that the treatment program is being handled with responsibility. If a person telephones in distress asking for help to handle a real-life situation aside from the pain, an appointment is given as soon as possible to reinforce the idea that asking for help is more responsible than converting that stress into pain in order to gain attention and help. For

instance, a person who had had a severe cervical pain problem tele-
phoned because of panic associated with university exams and was
given a prompt appointment, and the old pattern of slipping back
into neck pain was avoided. However, when a person telephones
only because of the pain, a delay in giving an appointment is necessary in order to avoid a close temporal association between the pain
behaviour of telephoning and reinforcement by attention. The pain
patient may need to be confronted with his dependent behaviour if
this occurs more than once. For instance, a patient with back pain
who refused to leave a medical consultant's surgery without a
promise of telephone counselling that evening was confronted with
her dependent behaviour and was given the option of continuing
treatment in an adult, responsible manner or being discharged. She
accepted the former, and has continued in the treatment situation
with considerable improvement in her family relationships and no
further mention of the back pain was undoubtedly psychogenic in
origin.

Handing the responsibility for further appointments to the person with pain avoids the development of dependency, does not give
rise to feelings of rejection by full discharge, and allows time for
changes to occur.

TREATMENT COMPONENTS

Assessment session

The first session allows the person with pain and the physiotherapist to assess each other. To work together in a successful partnership, mutual trust must develop. The therapist must be careful
not to allow the patient to move into a detailed monologue of symptoms that has been rehearsed thoroughly with previous therapists.
After showing initial interest in the pain site the therapist firmly
moves away from the discussion of the pain to a discussion of a
pain-pattern, which is used as a base for taking a history.

The initial history relates to stress with questions like the following:
'How frustrated/annoyed/irritated are you by the pain?'
'How worried do you get about it?'
'Chronic pain is a stressor—how do you handle other stresses in your life?'
'How did you learn to handle stress, i.e., how did your parents handle stress?'

After a simple explanation has been given of how the body reacts
to stress, in terms of flight, fight or freeze, the therapist may ask

where tension is noticed in the body when busy or pressured or angry or worried.

The therapist should have gained an impression of the person by what is being said and should be observing, also, the manner in which that person is sitting and using his body while talking. This type of interview usually is unexpected and will be generating some stress that may be showing non-verbally in body language. The person may be sitting on the edge of the chair, rocking, gripping the chair arms, sitting hunched up, sitting with the head thrust forward, or may be clenching the jaw and frowning. Gently, attention can be drawn to any such posture in order to make the point that the body is expressing something about the way the individual is feeling at that moment. Some explanation needs to be given of the manner in which stress is being shown in body language, in order to demonstrate the basic loop of the pain-pattern, i.e. 'pain causes stress that is expressed by the muscle system in such a way that pain is perpetuated'. The link between the mind and body, suffering and pain, will be starting to form.

Movement is then away from assessment and into treatment (Fig. 3.2), although in successive sessions further assessment of the development of the pain-pattern will continue along with treatment.

Education about pain

Patients have been taught and most firmly believe that all pain has an organic cause. When an organic cause appropriate to the symptoms has not been elicited, the patient has comprehended the message that the pain is not real or that he is malingering or attention-seeking or neurotic. Such messages, either overt or covert, increase the emotional reaction to the pain situation and so the basic loop of the pain-pattern is completed and pain increases. The patient who resists such messages probably will believe that there must be an undiagnosed organic cause and will imagine cancer, tumours or other malignant diseases; fear increases and so does the pain.

It is important, therefore, to teach the person with pain gradually that the word *pain* entails emotion and that pain does not necessarily have an organic base. Behaviour of the body can cause pain. This lesson about the nature of pain may need to be repeated many times before the subject will accept it fully as it is so strongly contrary to current belief systems.

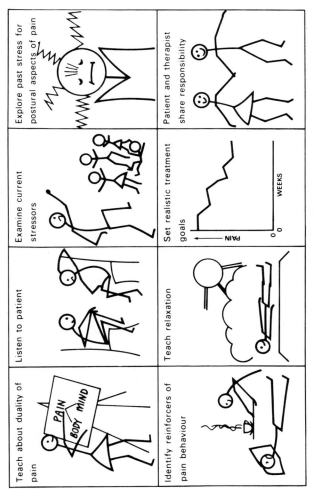

Fig. 3.2 Treat mind and body together to alleviate pain (poster, WCPT Congress, Stockholm, 1982).

Relaxation training

People with chronic pain usually will agree readily that the pain worries and irritates them. As relaxation is incompatible with both anxiety and irritability it is appropriate to introduce relaxation training in the initial sessions.

Verbal methods of relaxation training can be used. Jacobson's (1929) progressive relaxation training is a slow, repetitive, carefully assessed progression of orders that helps a subject to develop a muscle sense along with a sense of relaxation. Unfortunately, much teaching that purports to use this method tends to be a vigorous contrast between muscle tightening and letting go. The subtlety of the method is lost and excessive action will mask the very purpose of the therapist's observation: traces of the subject's muscle activity as a response to stress.

Physiological relaxation training (Mitchell, 1977) moves the body away from the fear posturing of flexion/adduction/elevation and draws attention to the perception of the new position.

Autogenic training (Luthe, 1971) focuses on the sensations that accompany relaxation by using a series of repetitive phrases.

A simple verbal routine focuses on body awareness and can be used for home practice or can be paired with biofeedback training. A script for this routine follows (see Appendix, page 70).

In order to transfer the learning and practice of relaxation away from the clinical situation, a cassette tape can be used for home practice. The therapist may be skilled enough to record the actual clinical relaxation training session so that home practice is based on a routine tailored to suit the needs of that particular individual.

Electromyographic biofeedback

Biofeedback relaxation

The advantage of biofeedback-mediated relaxation training over other methods is that an objective measure of the relaxation response is obtained.

The subject sits or lies in a fully supported position in which discomfort due to the pain is minimized — a pillow under the knees in lying will ease strain on the spine; a side-lying position with a pillow supporting the upper arm may ease chest pain.

Electrodes are placed on the forehead with the two active electrodes placed 1 inch above each eyebrow and the ground electrode in between. It should be noted that this electrode placement reflects a total or global electromyogram (EMG) of varied repeated, dynamic muscular activities down to about the first rib and is not 'frontalis EMG' (Basmajian, 1979).

EMG biofeedback measures vary due to technicalities involved in the rectification of the raw EMG. Using a bandwidth of 100–1000 Hz, amplitudes averaging around 0.5–1.0 microvolt seem to be typical of relaxed muscles in the forehead area, whereas headache sufferers may have readings as high as 10 microvolts (Peffer, 1979).

The nature of the recording instrument is explained and demonstrated to the subject and instructions are given to be aware of the tone and the manner in which it gradually lowers and settles. Attention to the tone should be passive, as active listening involving concentration will induce activity in the facial muscles. Recordings are taken over 15 minutes while the subject rests quietly.

Pairing the verbal body awareness relaxation routine with the audiofeedback can be a useful way to introduce the relaxation session. The voice of the therapist can be reassuring whereas the fluctuations of the tone may provoke anxiety in an already anxious subject. The verbal routine can be given in a way that suits the individual subject's needs, and will possibly not be needed once a routine for relaxation with feedback has become established.

After 15 minutes or so the tone is turned down and the subject is asked quietly to describe the sensations present in his body, as putting sensations into words helps to memorize those sensations.

A graph of EMG activity is drawn during each session so that behaviour within each session and across sessions can be demonstrated to and discussed with the subject (Fig. 3.3). The following information is obtained from the graphs.

1. *Level of EMG activity.* A mean around 1 microvolt is usually accompanied by subjective sensations of deep relaxation. A mean around 3 microvolts indicates rest rather than relaxation. A higher mean indicates either localized tension in the facial muscles or anxiety or irritability.

2. *Slope over time.* An upward slope indicates increasing anxiety while a downward slope indicates some ability to reduce muscle activity. The former is more likely to mean that the subject has to learn *how* to relax while the latter possibly means that the subject has to *allow* himself to relax.

3. *A restless pattern.* The subject may not be attending to the

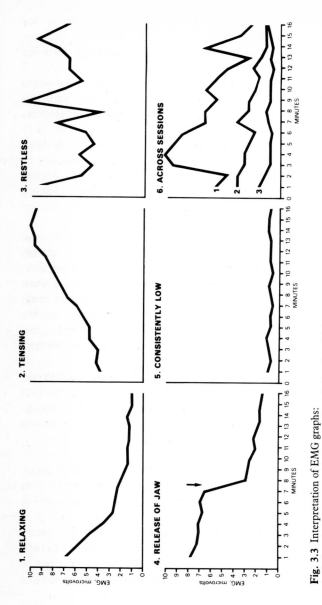

Fig. 3.3 Interpretation of EMG graphs:
1. Relaxation, low mean, downward slope 2. Tensing, high mean, upward slope 3. Restlessness 4. Release of jaw
5. Consistently low readings 6. Across sessions.

audiofeedback signal or relaxation training may not be appropriate at that moment.

4. *A sudden drop.* The subject may suddenly become aware of tension and may release it. This is marked, for example, when the subject becomes aware of clenching the teeth and suddenly lets the jaw drag down.

5. *A consistently low* recording of EMG may indicate complete relaxation but sometimes seems incompatible with the observed behaviour and the symptoms of the patient. Sometimes the social history indicates that the subject may have learned from a very early age not to allow any trace of emotion to show in the facial muscles.

6. *Across sessions.* Several sessions can be plotted on one set of axes allowing comparison and showing progress over time.

EMG analysis of muscle activity

When an animal is threatened it either attacks, runs away or freezes on the spot; each of these actions activates the entire muscle system. Human beings, when under threat, respond in the same manner, although social learning, for most people, has taught them almost always not to attack and under most conditions not to run away. Most people have been conscious at times of feeling frozen to the spot, of wishing 'the floor would open under them' to allow escape. Some people attack verbally rather than physically and others will not even allow themselves to do that.

Earlier, it was noted that chronic pain caused stress; it is a threat to the person as it prevents the fulfilment of tasks and the achievement of goals. When the person's muscle response to stress is superimposed on the pain site, the pain is perpetuated. EMG muscle analysis of this muscle activity can identify and be used to alter this pattern. Examples, based on clinical observation, follow.

1. *The forehead.* If the EMG drops abruptly when the instruction is given 'to smooth out the wrinkles and unfold the frowns' it is useful to look for *conflict* in the subject's life. Making a decision requires concentration and the forehead expression shows this. When circumstances make it impossible for that decision to be made so that a problem can be resolved, it seems probable that the muscles governing that expression remain in a state of contraction. If the therapist observes this pattern of forehead muscle behaviour it is useful to suggest that conflicts or unresolved problems are troublesome.

2. *The jaw.* Muscle action around the temporo-mandibular joint

can be monitored by placing the active electrodes above and below that joint; EMG readings should be taken with the subject sitting, standing and lying down. In sitting the control of this joint may be obvious and even in lying control may be retained. It may be very difficult to allow the jaw to loosen and may be uncomfortable to do so as the sensation is foreign. It may take practice to be able to loosen the jaw while keeping the lips closed.

People showing this behaviour often speak quietly and are gentle, kind, well-behaved people who literally, 'hold back angry words'. Metaphors abound in the English language to describe this behaviour: 'keep ones mouth shut', 'keep a stiff upper lip', 'keep the lips sealed', 'hold ones tongue', 'grip the teeth and carry on', 'grind on', and a cockney expression says to 'stop jawing'. This behaviour often is associated with facial and neck pain.

When dentures have not been inspected for years, or the teeth look very uneven, or there is numbness over the side of the face, ringing in the ears, or extreme tenderness over the temporo-mandibular joint is reported, a referral for assessment to a dentist experienced in oral surgery may be applicable.

3. *The shoulders*. EMG monitoring of the upper fibres of the trapezius muscle frequently shows that the shoulders are kept slightly elevated. This can be a defensive posture and can be visualized as feeling prepared and alert to fight. It can also be associated with tears and unresolved grief: when sobbing deeply the shoulders heave. Envisaging that same person stopping those shoulders from moving gives a subjective sensation of control around the shoulder girdle and upper spine. The effort of stopping a muscle from contracting when the stimulus for muscle contraction is present appears to cause fatigue. People showing this behaviour often have not worked through a bereavement and relaxing these muscles may, indeed, bring tears.

Breathing

Maladaptive breathing patterns are associated often with chest and 'heart' pains. When the temporo-mandibular area is controlled, breathing patterns may be disrupted.

'Heavy breathing' is associated with fear and danger, so hyperventilation should be noted. People 'hold their breath' when anxious or frightened. The therapist should watch for hyperventilation and breath holding when the subject with pain is walking, talking and lying relaxed. The asthma resting position of high side-lying, with the top leg supported well forward and the top arm supported on a pillow, should be used for relaxation as an optimal position for normal breathing.

People often are unaware that they are using their breathing to help control pain. Abnormal breathing is less efficient and will tend to produce further symptoms which may increase anxiety and compound the pain-pattern further.

Fitness program

Chronic pain saps the energy; people are inclined to do less and lose their fitness with a resulting loss of wellbeing. In the acute phase of pain, patients have been told to rest and are often still 'resting' years later! It is important to confront people with chronic pain with a choice: 'You can either have pain and be fit, or have pain and be unfit. The choice is yours.'

Some people have lost their confidence to move and are afraid that exercise will increase damage—they need encouragement to get started. They should nominate their own way of regaining fitness and their own program; the therapist should note this and reinforce it with interest. Total exercise is preferable to specific exercises and can be brisk walking, running or jogging, swimming or cycling.

Brisk walking has most advantages for the majority of people as it is safe and will not jar the spine as jogging may do. A walking routine can be carried out anywhere; the whole muscle system is used in a coordinated way. Walking gives a person time alone to think and dream—it gives him space away from other demands.

The subject is asked to nominate a circuit from where he lives, estimate its distance and make a commitment to walk that circuit, briskly, once a day for six days a week. When this distance can be accomplished comfortably and the fear of causing further damage has diminished, encouragement is given to increase the distance, or to increase the number of walks taken daily, with the aim of being able to walk 3–4 miles a day. Warning is given that discomfort and pain may increase initially, as indeed would happen for any person who was unfit.

People who formerly have enjoyed sport as a recreation should be encouraged to return to sport even if it means being a coach or administrator instead of an active participant. Allegiance may have to be changed to another sport; one woman who was an avid squash player, after a neck injury that damaged her right arm, changed to bowls which she learned to play left-handed. The social consequence of meeting new people helped her rehabilitation.

Massage

The physiotherapist is trained to use massage for its physiological effects and should also use it for psychological effects.
1. Massage can denote *caring*. When pain seems to be associated with grief, massage to the neck and shoulders may release much of the tension that is perpetuating the pain.
2. Massage can alter the *perception* of pain. Sensory input that is pleasant from a part of the body that always feels unpleasant and sore alters the perception of that part of the body. For instance, light, brisk, rapid finger tapping over the temporal and forehead areas of the headache patient can alleviate the headache (cf. Transcutaneous electrical nerve stimulation, TENS).
3. Massage can be *communication*. When a relationship between two people has deteriorated because of stress that may be pain-related, massage of one partner by the other can initiate positive communication in a meaningful, non-verbal manner. This applies particularly when considering the third meaning of 'pain' given by Szasz.
4. Children in pain love massage; it offers *security*.

Pain behaviour

In Western society, because the meaning of the word 'pain' is considered to be organic, pain behaviour has been reinforced strongly by medical attention. The more complex the problem the more interesting it becomes and the greater the reinforcement of the patient's submissive, subservient role. Care and consideration within the family can also reinforce pain behaviour, especially when normally care tends to be minimal within that family. Careful observation will identify these reinforcers which should be withdrawn from pain behaviour and reapplied to rehabilitative behaviour.

For instance, on arrival the therapist should show interest by asking, 'What have you achieved this week?' rather than, 'Where have you felt the pain?' The subject's own efforts to take responsibility should be noted with comments like, 'How good that you walked 400 yards', rather than, 'What a shame it hurt too much to walk the half mile'.

'Pain games' can be explained (see Shealy, 1976). The small

child will have a sore stomach when school is stressful, and everyone occasionally has a headache to avoid a meeting. The patient with chronic pain may do this persistently without awareness and people around may be pandering to this behaviour rather than risking upsetting that person and making the pain worse; they may be unable to break out of this pattern of behaviour. For this reason it can be useful to include the spouse and family in one treatment session to try and identify reinforcers of *pain behaviour* that could be withdrawn while introducing reinforcers of *rehabilitation behaviour*.

Counselling

Physiotherapists are not trained to counsel, but the nature of their work, one-to-one contact with patients, means that they are the recipients of many patients' anxieties and problems so that many therapists develop sound listening skills (Conine, 1976).

The technique may therefore be as follows:

1. Listen to the *whole* person, verbally and non-verbally.

2. Listen to the *real* message of distress, sadness, loneliness and frustration and not just to the 'recorded' message of 'the pain is here, and there, and doctor said this and did that and the pain moved here and the specialist said this . . .'.

3. *Attend* to the message from the whole person rather than collude with the patient that the pain *is* the whole message—only allow the subject to give the recorded message once and on further utterances move all attention away from it.

Too often, the message from the patient is, 'If you make the pain go away everything else will be all right', to which the therapist must reply, 'If you make some of the other things in your life all right, you will handle the pain situation better and it might even diminish as well.'

Feelings

Pain is perpetuated by tension and this tension reflects irritability and anxiety. These feelings must be expressed and can usually be elicited by such comments as, 'You must be fed up with the pain', or, 'You must be worried about all that is happening to you'.

Often, there is a lot of anger about previous failed treatment approaches and it is important that people with pain should feel safe enough to be able to be angry about previous therapists and doctors who have build up their expectations for cure and disappointed them, or who have given messages implying that there is nothing really wrong. The therapist should listen to the feeling being expressed and not to the specific message about colleagues as nothing is to be gained by blaming others. Once this anger has been expressed the person with pain will often come to accept the reality that others have not been able to take the responsibility for his pain and that, indeed, he must take that responsibility himself.

Much anxiety about pain reflects other family experiences; someone may have had a stroke after headaches, or may have died from an undiagnosed tumour or have had cancer. It is important, if such fears are present, to arrange for examination by a medical specialist to eliminate the source of this anxiety. Once such fears are refuted, the person with pain may be able to see that it was his own anxious behaviour of, say, clenching the jaw in an act of stoicism that was producing facial pain. Alternatively, the person may be able to cry for the relation who died of cancer and by experiencing the grief the cervical pain might ease.

Self-esteem is often low, particularly if the belief is held that the pain is neurotic or hypochondriacal. It becomes necessary to identify aspects of the person's life that are satisfying and reinforce these with praise, e.g., 'In spite of your illness and pain your children are doing well at school; how well you are doing as a mother', or, 'As you have been promoted at work your employer must see you as a responsible person'.

A sense of humour helps many people to cope with stress but with chronic pain there is not much fun in life. If a person can learn to laugh, even when part of his body hurts, then he is well on the way to handling his problems more effectively.

The family

The family have often been left out of the scene and should be brought into the treatment scene, as chronic pain effects the whole family and the family, indeed, may be reinforcing pain behaviour. The family can provide useful information. They are useful allies in enforcing the treatment program and giving them this task may relieve their anxiety as at last they can help in some way; one family member may be a companion on walks and another may offer massage (for some in return!) They may become interested in observing their own and each other's behaviour in response to stress, and communication may increase.

The job

Counselling may centre around the job. Pain may result in a decision about a necessary change of job in a manner that induces conflict and stress. If the individual is off work there may be considerable anxiety about returning to work. Income may be reduced and it may be appropriate to refer to a budgeting service agency. In times of an economic recession a person may be forced to stay in a job that is unsuitable and may need support to be able to accept this. An ergonomic assessment of that job situation may be useful. Sometimes, a person aspires to a change of job and the pain problem gives the opportunity to make that change.

CAUTIONS

The physiotherapist would do well to adhere to these cautionary guidelines.

1. Work as a member of a team. The problems associated with pain are complex and may be solved best if several people work on them together. Keep in touch with the referring doctor.

2. Refer to other professional people when indicated. If many personal problems are present refer to a psychologist; if pressures are social or job-related the social worker may be more appropriate; if depression is severe a psychiatric assessment may be necessary; with facial pain a dental or oral surgeon may be able to help.

3. Remember that when a person relaxes he is no longer on guard; the defense system is lowered and he may disclose much information that he would not normally discuss. Treat such confidentiality with respect.

4. If a person shares deep and painful feelings and is distressed, make sure he has recovered sufficiently before allowing him to go home. Sometimes the subject is in a state of shock and a cup of coffee may help. If necessary, contact a family member to ensure support on return home, and if in doubt discuss the situation with the family doctor.

5. When the pain is communicative, in the third sense of Szasz, it may not be wise to remove that pain. Sometimes, if the spouse seems to be a negative person it may become apparent that the pain is the means by which one person in the relationship gives or obtains care. The pain may be necessary to uphold the relationship. Removal of the pain would be disastrous to that relationship and to other dependent relationships and would entail more responsi-

bility than that for which the physiotherapist is trained. A referral for psychiatric assessment should be made.

6. Note that this article is not definitive, as research and new clinical approaches are rapidly providing many new facts and ideas. Keep reading the literature.

CLINICAL EXAMPLES

The effectiveness of relaxation training as a skill to handle his lower back pain gave a man (42-year-old) confidence. In 10 months off work since a fall he had been seen by many people and was particularly angry with his own doctor and with psychiatrists. On his fourth visit he spoke of the death, 15 years previously, of his fiancé due to terrorist action in Northern Ireland. He had told no one of her death, only that the engagement was off. He married some years later, emigrated and worked hard to establish his family. The accident gave him time to himself and the grief, of which he was unaware, showed as depression and anger. After a total of 8 sessions, during which time he shared the grief with his wife, he was able to return to work. By separating the pain problem from the grief problem, although still sad and with a vulnerable back, he was able to take responsibility for his situation.

A girl of 18 was seen on twelve occasions over three months, for treatment for a recurrence of ankle pain that she had had a year previously after a fall. She had used crutches for months and had received much specialist attention. She looked unhappy and seemed to be at the centre of her parents' discord, and during the time of treatment her mother left home. She was employed by her father, was studying extramurally for her University Entrance exam that she had failed twice, and was managing the house and three younger siblings. Prior to being seen she had been physically attacked by her mother and said that she was very frightened and always sat near the door with her crutches between her and her mother. Treatment was supportive, with all attention taken away from the ankle. She needed the crutches at home for defence, but was encouraged, while out of the home, to walk without them. After her mother left she walked normally, passed her exams and was accepted for a training course in another city. She came to realise that, although she had a vulnerable ankle, it was other factors in her life that were preventing it from getting better.

A woman of 43 had severe facial pain following tooth extraction 10 months previously. Localised EMG monitoring showed high resting tension around the TMJ region, which she learned to relax. She shared anger about all that had happened and talked of having been afraid of her suicidal thoughts. She shared guilt about pain that her daughter had experienced two years previously which she had tended to dismiss lightly and which eventually proved very serious. This daughter was behaving badly and resented her mother's pain. Discussion with the daughter improved the relationship and the mother felt considerable relief and regained confidence, which led to her compliance with a regime of medication of which she had previously been suspicious. She had complete relief of pain, after nine sessions.

Phantom limb pain was severe for a man who lost his hand in an industrial accident. His physical recovery had been excellent and he returned to his old job, having mastered a prosthesis, within three months. Psychotherapy allowed him to recall the moment of the accident dramatically with insight into the nature of the pain; it was the press falling on the hand and he had a total recall of that moment. He was depressed after this and his wife, although unhappy, felt more able to support him through this than she had been able to in the earlier stoicism. Meanwhile, some therapy entailed work on the body image, general relaxation to decrease anxiety about the pain and specific localized EMG biofeedback on the residual ends of muscles in the forearm. These muscles would still contract when movement was initiated and because there was no proprioception due to the missing hand, these bits of muscle would go into spasm. Learning to contract and relax these muscle ends gave the sensation of altering the position of the phantom hand in such a manner that he could, with much concentration, alter the sensation of the position of the hand with a decrease in pain. Education about phantom limb pain and perception was important as later he admitted that he had thought he was going mad when he experienced extracorporeal pain. When last contacted this man had returned to playing golf, and although the pain was still present at times he was no longer overwhelmed by it and was happy. He was seen for 19 sessions, two with his wife.

APPENDIX: BODY AWARENESS RELAXATION ROUTINE

Sit back comfortably in a chair, or lie down, so your body is well supported . . . look around you . . . close your eyes quietly to shut out distractions. Listen to the sounds around you and identify them. If you identify the sounds they will not intrude. Now be very aware of the support for your body . . . feel the contact with that support, feel that it is *safe* enough to allow your body to ease. Now notice your breathing — not to change it, but just to feel the rhythm . . . see if you can feel yourself letting go a little each time you breathe out.

There are lots of sensations in the body that one does not usually attend to, and I am going to draw your attention to some of these. There is nothing right or wrong about how your body feels—just become aware of it.

First, notice your feet . . . be aware of how they feel when resting . . . now notice your knees, feel yourself allowing the knees to ease off . . . feel the contact between your hips and the chair or bed . . . feel how the support takes the weight of the hips and notice all the sensations around your hips.

Feel the position of your back on the support . . . you can feel how your spine curves and the pressures along your back vary . . . absorb the feeling of the support for your back . . . feel how safe it is to let go.

Now be aware of the position of your arms . . . especially the hands which are very sensitive. You can feel where each finger is . . . what it is touching . . . you can feel the texture of what the hands are touching. Sometimes, you can imagine the air on the skin of the hands . . . the skin is very sensitive.

Feel the angle of your elbows . . . when the elbows are supported you can feel the shoulders dropping a little . . . be aware of how the shoulders and the top of the chest loosen up a little each time you breathe out.

Now feel the support for your head . . . if it is on a pillow feel how the pillow takes the weight of the head so that the neck can ease. Feel the neck letting go.

Be aware of your face . . . see if you can capture the feeling that you don't need to keep a certain look on your face . . . the expression can drop into a neutral, resting position. Particularly notice your jaw . . . let it sag a little . . . feel the teeth separate a little, the opposite to gritting your teeth. When the jaw is loose, the cheeks are soft.

Notice your eyes. Sometimes the eyes themselves feel as if they are jumping around . . . imagine them in a neutral position. See if you can capture the sensation of the eyelids dropping by their own weight . . . there is no effort in holding them shut.

Now focus on your forehead — feel yourself unfolding your wrinkles . . . smoothing out the frowns. Just as you are aware of your body, be aware now of your thinking. There is nothing right or wrong about your thinking . . . just notice whether it is busy or calm . . . whether it is jumping around or flowing . . . allow it to do what it wants to do.

Now I shall stop talking, and I want you to lie quietly for a few minutes, enjoying the feeling of allowing yourself to rest quietly . . .

ACKNOWLEDGEMENT

Acknowledgement is made to the Medical Illustrations Department, Christchurch Hospital, Christchurch, N.Z., for permission to use the illustrations in this chapter.

REFERENCES

Arbogast R C, Huffer V 1978 Current concepts in psychosomatic medicine: biofeedback. Maryland State Medical Journal 27: 59–61
Baier J 1970 In: Trigg R (ed) Pain and emotion. Clarendon Press.
Basmajian J V 1978 Muscles alive, 4th edn. Williams and Wilkins, Baltimore
Beecher H K 1966 Pain: one mystery solved. Science 151: 840–841
Bobey M J, Davidson P O 1970 Psychological factors affecting pain tolerance. Journal of Psychosomatic Research 14: 371–376
Cassell E J 1982 The nature of suffering and the goals of medicine. The New England Journal of Medicine 306: 11: 639–645
Conine T A 1976 Listening in a helping relationship. Physical Therapy S6: 159–162
Cox T 1978 Stress. University Park Press, Baltimore Md.
Fordyce W E, Fowler R S, Lehmann J F, DeLateur B J, Sand P L, Trieschmann R B 1973 Operant conditioning in the treatment of chronic pain. Archives of Physical Medicine and Rehabilitation 54: 399–407
Grzesiak R C 1977 Relaxation techniques in the treatment of chronic pain. Archives of Physical Medicine and Rehabilitation 58: 270–272
Hendler N 1977 EMG biofeedback in patients with chronic pain. Diseases of the Nervous System 505–509
Jacobson E 1929 Progressive relaxation. University of Chicago Press, Chicago
Leavitt F, Garron D C, Whisler W W, Sheinkop M B 1978 Affective and Sensory dimensions of back pain. Pain 4: 273–281
Luthe W 1971 Autogenic therapy. In: Biofeedback and Self Control 437–473
Melzack R 1973 The puzzle of pain. Basic Books, New York
Melzack R, Torgerson W S 1971. On the language of pain. Anesthesiology 34: 50–59
Mitchell L 1977 Simple relaxation. John Murray, London
Moon M H 1982a Post-operative pain, EMG biofeedback measures and relaxation. Proceedings IXth International Congress of Physical Therapy. Sweden
Moon M H 1982b Psychology of pain. Proceedings IXth International Congress of Physical Therapy, Sweden
Older J 1983 Review of Under the Doctor, New Zealand Journal of Physiotherapy 11:1:33

Peffer K E 1978 Equipment needs for the psychotherapist. In: Basmajian J (ed) Biofeedback: principles and practices for clinicians. Williams and Wilkins, Baltimore

Ryle G 1968 In: Cowan J L (ed) Pleasure and pain: a study: philosophical psychology. MacMillan, London

Schwartz G E, Fair P L, Salt P, Mandel M R, Klerman G L 1976 Facial expression and imagery in depression: an electromyographic study. Psychosomatic Medicine 38: 5: 337–347

Selye H 1975 Stress without distress. Hodder and Stoughton, London

Shealy C N 1976 The pain game. Celestial Arts, California

Szasz T S 1957 Pain and pleasure. Tavistock, London

Turk D C, Meichenbaum D H, Berman W H 1979 Application of biofeedback for the regulation of pain. Psychological Bulletin 86: 6: 1322–1338

Wickramaskera I 1972 EMG feedback training and tension headache. American Journal of Clinical Hypnosis 15: 83–85

TENS: uses and effectiveness

What is TENS?

Transcutaneous electrical nerve stimulation (TENS) means the transmission of electrical energy across the surface of the skin to the nervous system. Electricity is a natural phenomenon within all types of living tissue. The brain constantly receives and integrates electrical signals indicative of all environmental (external) and bodily (internal) events including that of pain.

One type of electrical impulse that can signal impending damage, merely annoy, partially hinder or totally incapacitate is the impulse of nociception. The nociceptive impulse mediating the sensation of pain is also a prime impetus that brings the patient to a health practitioner.

Throughout history man has sought relief from pain by various means. Historical references to pain-relieving modalities include herbs, potions, heat and cold applications, acupuncture techniques, drugs, surgery, meditation, hypnosis and electricity. TENS incorporates an early method of pain relief that has now been refined and simplified for ease of application via the use of new scientific and technological advances.

Historical references to the use of electricity to decrease or control pain begin in the year 46 A.D. when a Roman physician, Scribonius Largus, described how the electric stimulus for a Torpedo fish (electric eel) was able to provide pain relief for headache and gout (Hymes, 1984; Taub and Kane, 1975). One of the first commercially available TENS devices that was battery powered and touted for pain control, among many other indications, appeared in 1919 and was known as the 'Electreat' (Barcalow, 1919) In its original design the Electreat had only one adjustable parameter, amplitude, with pulse rate and width being fixed. The device produces a strong electrical paresthesia and is still in use in its original form.

Publication of Melzack and Wall's gate control theory in 1965 produced a reawakening of scientists and clinicians involved in pain research and management (Melzack & Wall, 1965). Based upon the original tenets of this theory, that has since been reviewed and analyzed by many (Wolf, 1984). Shealy and Mortimer developed a stimulator that transmitted electrical impulses to surgically implanted electrodes over the dorsal columns of the spinal cord in 1967 (Shealy et al, 1967; Shealy & Mortimer, 1970). This device became known as the dorsal column stimulator (DCS) and was used exclusively for patients with chronic intractable pain.

DCS usage spawned the development of TENS devices in the early 1970s as transcutaneous electrodes were used to evaluate patients as good candidates for a DCS. A significant number of patients obtained satisfactory pain control with TENS thus fostering its initial development.

TENS devices are now being manufactured by many companies in various countries. It is estimated that in the United States alone at least 30 manufacturers produce their own TENS units. International manufacturers exist in Canada, England, France, Sweden, Germany, Russia, China, Japan and Israel. Similar portable electrical stimulators use invasive electrodes placed either around a peripheral nerve over the dorsal columns of the spinal cord or within various brain-stem sites. These stimulators thus differ from TENS units and are known as percutaneous (PCS), dorsal column (DCS) and deep brain (DBS) stimulators respectively (Ray, 1977). The electrodes that are utilized with these electrical stimulators require surgical implantation, thus taking them out of the realm of the physical therapist.

A TENS unit is small, portable, battery powered and specifically designed for use by the patient at home. It thus becomes a modern alternative to drugs of both the narcotic and non-narcotic variety. In the United States it is available only upon physician prescription but in Japan it can be purchased over the counter.

TENS and medication

TENS, like medicinal applications, may relieve part or all of a patient's pain for varying periods of time. However, the use of TENS is not governed by specific time intervals like medication in which dosages may, for example, be taken only once every four hours. There is no limit to the number of stimulation periods in a given day in which TENS can be used. TENS can thus provide sustained pain relief whereas medication will wax and wane in benefit as its effect wears off and a period of time must elapse before another dose can be taken. There are many side-effects which can occur from medicinal use, especially of the narcotic variety. Apart from the possibility of addiction, narcotics may cause such effects as pruritis, cutaneous vasodilation, constipation, respiratory depression, lethargy, and a loss of mental acuity. Utilization of TENS will not cause any of the aforementioned side-effects but a small percentage of patients (less than 2%) may develop an allergic reaction to the electrode, its transmission medium or tape patch (Fisher, 1978). Improper utilization of TENS can cause skin irritation in the form of erythema or actual burns of the pin-point variety or blistering and tissue damage. This usually occurs from improper placement of the electrodes, sparse application of transmission gel or pre-gelled electrodes that dry out. High frequency pulse rates are more likely to produce skin irritation than low frequency pulse rates. TENS, unlike medication, is difficult to use with a senile or aphasic patient and those with visual or hand dysfunction may have difficulty operating the device.

The positive effects of narcotics, besides pain relief, are sedation and mood enhancement. In comparison, TENS can provide sustained pain control along with continuous mental acuity that can allow for active patient participation in home or hospital therapeutic sessions. The use of TENS post-operatively highlights the value of patient participation.

Indications, contraindications and precautions

TENS can be used adjunctively as a symptomatic means of pain control in a wide variety of acute, chronic and post-surgical conditions. Whenever a physician prescribes medication for pain relief there are but a few reasons why TENS cannot be used in lieu of such medication. The only absolute contraindication to the use of TENS is in the presence of a demand-type cardiac pacemaker. The electrical impulse produced by TENS may interfere with the action of the pacemaker (Shealy & Maurer, 1974; Ericksson et al, 1978). TENS may also interfere with encephalographic and cardiac monitors. However, filtering devices are easily manufactured that can interface between the TENS device and the monitor (Peper & Grimbergen, 1983; Furno & Tompkins, 1983).

There are specific precautions when using TENS which relate primarily to the area of electrode placement. Electrodes should not be placed directly on the eye. However, transcutaneous and sub-cutaneous electrodes have been successfully positioned on the supra and infraorbital regions for pain control after eye surgery without any negative effects (Ticho et al, 1980). The following precautions should be considered when the use of TENS is contemplated:

1. Stimulation in the area of the carotid sinus nerves may produce laryngeal and/or pharyngeal spasm effecting blood pressure and respiration.

2. Stimulation over superficial aspects of bone such as the forehead and tibial shaft may not be tolerated well. The periosteum is highly innervated and is thus very sensitive to even mild stimulation.

3. Care must be taken when TENS is employed near or over the heart in patients with myocardial disease. The electrical energy produced by a TENS unit however, is not enough to cause cardiac fibrillation (Shealy & Maurer, 1974). When used in the presence of cardiac disease it is recommended that only a mild stimulation mode, known as conventional, be used and muscle contractions should not occur.

4. Caution is suggested when TENS is used on the head or neck in patients with epilepsy, transient ischemic attacks (TIA) or those who have had a cerebrovascular accident (CVA). It is possible, although not documented, that TENS may trigger an epileptic seizure when stimulation is provided in this area. Certain stimulation parameters or programmed modes can produce significant vasodilation and may trigger detrimental vascular effects in patients with a history of TIA or a CVA.

5. The use of TENS during pregnancy is also considered to be precautionary. The effect on the unborn fetus is relatively unknown. However, TENS has been used successfully for pain control during labour and delivery (Augustinsson et al, 1977; Bundsen & Ericksson, 1982). Electrode placement in this instance is at T10–L1 and S2–S4 via paraspinally placed rectangular electrodes for control of stage one and stage two labor pain respectively. Bundsen recommends placement of a pair of electrodes over the groin and lower abdominal region for the second stage of labor in addition to the S2–S4 placement. There have not been any harmful effects noted to the fetus or the newborn (Augustinsson et al, 1977; Bundsen & Ericksson, 1982). During pregnancy TENS can be placed in areas other then the abdomen as long as only the mild conventional stimulation mode is used. Muscle contractions must be avoided. In this form TENS is equivalent to that of a superficial

massage in terms of intensity and depth of penetration. I have successfully used TENS for control of cervical and lumbar spine pain, post auto-accident in two women who were in the third trimester of pregnancy. Electrodes were placed paraspinally via separate channels at the cervical and lumbar regions. TENS was used at home in lieu of medication and both women had normal deliveries and healthy babies.

The adjunctive role of TENS in pain management

TENS must be considered as an adjunctive modality within the framework of a comprehensive rehabilitation program for the patient with acute or chronic pain. A comprehensive program is one which consists of a thorough patient evaluation, specific treatment geared to correction of the dysfunctional structure or removal of irritation, pain control and prophylaxis to prevent recurrence. TENS can only assist in one phase of such a program, namely that concerned with pain control (Mannheimer & Lampe, 1984a). TENS should therefore not be considered a treatment modality. It does not treat anything but merely serves as a means of symptomatic relief and/or control of discomfort. Unfortunately, to the detriment of the medical profession, the modality itself and also the patient, TENS has been severly abused. It is quite common to hear of situations in which the sole treatment for various types of pain, regardless of the cause, has been TENS. Furthermore, such treatment is frequently provided solely in the clinic on a periodic basis without any use of the device at home by the patient. The utilization of TENS in this manner is in no way comprehensive and treatment is only symptomatic in nature.

Treatment that consists entirely of TENS on a three-times per week basis in the clinic should be equated with having a patient report to the clinic at the same frequency for two aspirins and a glass of water after which he may lie down on a plinth for 30 minutes! TENS must not replace definitive therapy that treats, restores function and relieves irritation as opposed to just controlling discomfort. Optimal effectiveness with TENS occurs when it is used by the patient at home, while specific treatment is provided in the clinic setting.

There is a distinct role for the use of TENS in the clinic when it is needed to relieve and/or control pain prior to, during or after the performance of specific therapeutic procedures (Mannheimer

& Lampe, 1984a; Mannheimer, 1980; Mannheimer, 1983; Mannheimer & Lampe, 1984b). Techniques such as joint mobilization, contract–relax stretching, transverse friction massage and skin debridement are commonly painful to the patient. TENS can be used to allow for the performance by the therapist of the aforementioned procedures, providing adherence to specific safety guidelines are followed which will be presented later on in this chapter. There are also instances in which TENS may be the only viable modality that can be administered to the patient. Patients with pain syndromes such as trigeminal neuralgia, herpes zoster (shingles) and discomfort from severe functional changes due to rheumatoid or osteo-arthritis may obtain satisfactory pain relief from TENS when nothing else is helpful.

The initial indication for TENS in the early 1970s was as a last resort modality for the patient with chronic pain. After all forms of medical intervention such as medication, physical therapy, psychotherapy, and surgery had failed, TENS was prescribed. Only 25–50% of such chronic pain patients obtained satisfactory pain relief with TENS. If TENS is able to provide pain relief that is satisfactory to the patient and equal to or better than that obtained with medication I consider the result to be positive. Clinical results now confirm that the greatest degree of efficacy with TENS is achieved when it is instituted early in the acute stage of pain. Satisfactory results with TENS as a means of pain control in acute pain patients is better than 80%. It is a rare occurrence when I am unable to obtain satisfactory pain control with patients who have sustained acute cervical or lumbar strains, tendinitis and other musculoskeletal injuries. The use of TENS in the acute stage is of course dependent upon early referral by the physician. Comprehensive rehabilitation programs which include the use of TENS at home can significantly decrease the development of chronicity.

THE TENS SYSTEM

A TENS device is about the size of a pack of cigarettes and thus easily worn by the patient via a belt clip. The unit consists of electrical circuitry powered by one or more batteries that produce and transmit electrical impulses to the skin via lead wire cables and surface electrodes. Batteries may be either of the alkaline, lithium or nickel-cadmium rechargeable variety.

TENS units generate electrical impulses in specific waveforms. The TENS waveform must be balanced in that a net positive or negative direct current (DC) potential does not occur. A galvanic effect from an unbalanced waveform can produce skin irritations and discomfort thus negating the repetitive usage that is required by many pain patients. The most common waveform is therefore termed biphasic which may also be called faradic or alternating current (AC). The positive and negative components need not be identical in shape as viewed on an oscilloscope. Asymmetrical biphasic waveforms can also be balanced and equal in energy. The amount of energy per pulse is a product of the amplitude (intensity) plus the pulse width (duration). Increasing or decreasing either parameter will alter the strength of the pulse.

The critical determinant of effective stimulation is not the shape of the waveform but the electrical parameters that the unit can generate. In order to be effective a TENS unit must be capable of generating electrical energy sufficient to cause depolarization of the appropriate peripheral nerve. Sub-threshold stimulation, although helpful in patients with neuropathies or areas where there is hyperesthesia, is not considered to be significantly better than relief obtained by placebo administration (Thorsteinsson et al, 1978; Long et al, 1979; Andersson, 1979). Standards for labeling, safety and performance requirements for TENS devices has been developed by the Association for the Advancement of Medical Instrumentation (AAMI 1981).

The adjustable stimulation parameters are amplitude, measured in milliamps (mA), pulse duration measured in microseconds (μs) and pulse frequency or rate measured in cycles or pulses per second and expressed in terms of hertz (Hz). TENS units are available in single or dual channel formats. Dual channel units are much more common today and offer greater versatility in the management of two areas of pain or pain that is distributed through an extensive area. Single channel units may merely have an adjustable amplitude control or offer adjustment of two or all three parameters. Dual channel units with minimal manual adjustments offer independent amplitude controls per channel and at least a common pulse rate and pulse duration control. Common pulse rate and duration controls effect both channels simultaneously. Dual channel units are also available which offer independent pulse width and/or pulse rate controls per channel.

Stimulation parameters

Stimulation parameters, if adjustable, commonly fall within the following range for the majority of manufacturers: amplitude 0–80 mA, pulse rate 1–150 Hz and pulse duration 30–250μs. The clinician can program a variety of stimulation modes with different adjustments of these parameters. Newer models offered by many manufacturers also provide for controls that may interrupt or burst the programmed parameters (burst or pulse-train stimulation) or modulate (fluctuate) one or more parameters. Devices that offer the clinician all of the aforementioned features are the most sophisticated units available.

Electrode cables (lead wires)

Electrode cables (lead wires) allow for the transmission of the electrical impulses from the stimulator to the electrodes. Electrode cables are available in various lengths and are usually color coded to denote channel separation and/or polarity. Each channel may have a common receptacle for a dual lead wire cable or offer two receptacles for single lead wires one of which is positive, the other negative. Cable bifurcators commonly known as 'Y' adaptors allow for the use of more than two electrodes per channel. Electrode cables terminate in either a pin or snap connector for attachment to the electrodes. Adaptors are also available to convert pin leads to snap leads for added versatility.

Electrodes

The most common material used to manufacture transcutaneous electrodes is carbon-silicone. These electrodes are available in various sizes and shapes, most frequently square, rectangular or circular. A transmission medium is required as an interface between the electrode and the skin. Various conductive gels are available for this purpose and require hand application to thoroughly coat the surface of the electrode that lies against the skin. Pre-gelled electrodes are also available in different sizes, are self-adherent and may be used for approximately 1–5 days without being removed.

Natural and synthetic polymer materials that are both conductive and adhesive are also available as an electrode interface. Karaya is a natural polysaccharide that is used in the manufacture of many types of self-adhering electrodes.* Karaya is available in different degrees of thickness and thus varying amounts of impedance (re-

---

* Lec-tec Corp. 10205 Crosstown Circle, Eden Prairie, Minnesota. 55344

sistance to electrical transmission). Aquapore^{TM} is a new interface material that is 95% water with a very low impedence.**

The neurophysiologic basis to the development of the stimulation modes

A knowledge of the sensory changes and physiological effects associated with manipulation of each stimulation parameter is essential for the clinician to explain to the patient the sensation to expect with TENS. Amplitude and pulse duration settings determine the total energy per pulse. As the total amount of energy progresses, a greater number of nerve fibers are recruited, the sensation becomes stronger and the depth of stimulus penetration increases. The amount of energy per pulse further determines whether or not muscle contractions will occur. The pulse rate setting if below 10–15 Hz allows for the sensation of individual pulses or muscle contractions but if the rate exceeds 15–20 Hz electrical paresthesia or a tingling sensation occurs.

The normal human nervous system is easily able to perceive the sensation of each individual pulse as long as the frequency remains below 10–15 Hz. When the frequency exceeds 20 Hz the nervous system has greater difficulty separating the sensation of each pulse and, as a result, a merging of pulses occurs producing a constant electrical paresthesia. Various combinations of stimulation parameters can result in the production of an infinite amount of minor or major sensory changes.

A combination of low frequency (1–10 Hz) and low pulse energy (1–15 mA, 30–50 μs) may be below the perception threshold or produce a sensation of mild rhythmic pulsing without muscle contraction or fasciculation. Low frequency (1–10 Hz) and high pulse energy (30–60 mA, 150–200 μs) will cause strong rhythmic muscle contractions. Parameter settings of 50–100 Hz with a mild to moderate amount of pulse energy (15–30 mA, 50–150 μs) results in a continuous and comfortable electrical paresthesia. If the pulse energy is further increased upwards to 60 mA and 200 μs, strong electrical paresthesia and muscle tetany will occur. Non-rhythmic muscle fasciculation may also occur if full tetany is not obtained or fatigue sets in. A complete description of the sensations and physiologic effects that occur with changes solely of one stimulation

** Biostim Inc. Clarksville Road and Everett Drive, P.O. Box 3138, Princeton, New Jersey 08540

parameter while the other two are fixed is available from other publications (Mannheimer & Lampe, 1984c; Biostim Inc, 1983).

The aforementioned examples of parameter combinations and their resultant sensory effects may be minimized or maximized by other factors such as the interelectrode distance, electrode size, impedence and electrode placement sites. As the distance between two electrodes of one channel decreases less pulse energy is required to produce the desired sensation or effect. An increase in the interelectrode distance proportionately increases the amount of pulse energy necessary for the desired results. Lead wire bifurcators used to increase the number of electrodes per channel also result in the need for a greater degree of pulse energy.

The smaller the electrode, the greater the current density beneath it: smaller electrodes therefore require less pulse energy to produce the sensory and motor effects obtained with larger electrodes. The higher the impedance of the electrode and its interface as well as the underlying skin the greater the amount of pulse energy needed to produce the desired effect. Dry scaly skin has a great deal of resistance to electricity and electrode placement at these areas is not recommended. Electrode placement sites at areas where there are acupuncture, motor or trigger points as well as superficial peripheral nerve branches offer greater electrical conductance and lower impedance than areas which are not so densely innervated (Mannheimer, 1978; Mannheimer, 1980; Mannheimer & Lampe, 1984d). The greater the depth of the peripheral nerve from the skin surface and stimulating electrode the greater the impedance between the two. The excitablity characteristics of nerve fibers further provides scientific basis for the different stimulation modes. Basic neurophysiologic tenets state that myelineated nerve fibers conduct an electrical impulse at a faster velocity than non-myelinated fibers (Sinclair, 1981). In addition, the larger the diameter of the fiber the more rapid is its conduction velocity. Larger diameter fibers also contain a greater volume of axoplasm which is easily excitable. Therefore, the largest myelinated afferent nerve fibers (A alpha and beta) are the most rapid conducting (40–120 M/sec) and also the easiest to excite or depolarize.

The direct opposite in conduction and excitability characteristics are the nonmyelineated C fibers. These fibers are very thin, lack a myelin sheath and thus conduct very slowly at a speed that does not exceed 2–3 M/sec (Sinclair, 1981). C fibers have a smaller volume of axoplasm and require a greater amount of pulse energy for excitation or depolarization.

A alpha and beta fibers mediate afferent information pertaining to touch, proprioception and kinesthesis (Sinclair, 1981). A gamma fibers convey information relative to changes in muscle length. A delta fibers, the smallest of the myelineated A fibers, mediate nociceptive information primarily related to superficial, sharp, easy to localize pain. C fibers mediate nociceptive information more indicative of deep, achy, hard to localize pain of the chronic variety.

A knowledge of the aforementioned neurophysiologic factors as well as mechanisms relative to a variety of pain syndromes is necessary to gain an understanding for the programming and administration of TENS. Based on the Gate Control Theory of Pain (Melzack & Wall, 1965), inputs from large proprioceptive fibers provide a balancing effect to small nociceptive fiber input at the dorsal horn of the spinal cord (Melzack & Wall, 1965; Wolf, 1984; Sinclair, 1981; Mannheimer & Lampe, 1984e; Wolf et al, 1981). This is easily understood when one considers the effects which occur following a simple ankle sprain. If the individual who sustains an ankle sprain assumes a non-weight bearing position and does nothing to soothe the discomfort or distract his attention from the injured area, input from small nociceptive fibers predominates. This nociceptive input resulting from tissue damage and edema disrupts the normal dorsal horn input. Since there is no active or passive ankle movement, touch, temperature change (heat or cold application) or mental stimulation in the form of music, television or conversation, stimuli conducive to proprioceptive input is non-existent and pain predominates. However, if the injured area is gently massaged, mobilized, treated with cryotherapy or mental distraction provided, pain perception will be decreased. These forms of stimuli provide large afferent fiber input.

The stimulation modes

A significant amount of the material presented in this section is adapted from a previous publication by myself specifically comparing the characteristics and role of the different stimulation modes (Mannheimer, 1983). Pain syndromes differ via their neurophysiologic mechanisms and the resultant quality, depth, intensity and distribution of discomfort. The quality of pain that a patient perceives may also be indicative of involvement of more than one tissue structure. Pain arising from an arthritic joint is an excellent example. The quality of pain which stems from the synovial joint can thus be representative of each distinct structure which acts upon the joint. Furthermore, various tissue structures have different types and degrees of afferent innervation producing variations in pain quality and distribution. TENS units should therefore be capable of generating different stimulation modes to excite either a selective type or the full range of nerve fibers for the widest possible efficacy.

Recent clinical and technological advances have led to the development of four distinctly different stimulation modes: conventional, strong low rate (acupuncturelike), pulse-train (burst) and brief-intense. Alternations of these modes by forms of parameter modulation allow for programming of an infinite variety of sensory and motor stimuli.

Conventional

The stimulation modes differ significantly by many factors such as parameter settings, depth of tissue penetration, electrode placement techniques, speed of action, duration of pain relief and physiological effects. When TENS units first became commercially available in the early 1970s manufacturer recommendations were for stimulation parameter settings to deliver only a mild, low intensity and high frequency sensation which has come to be known as the conventional mode of TENS.

The conventional mode which has a wide range of clinical application is not universally effective for all pain syndromes or each patient in a group with a similar pain syndrome. The clinician who becomes familiar with and evaluates the efficacy of other stimulation modes will be able to enhance the effectiveness of TENS. Although two or more stimulation modes may be beneficial for a specific patient or pain syndrome one mode will usually provide greater pain relief that may also be longer lasting (Mannheimer & Lampe, 1984b; Mannheimer & Lampe, 1984c).

The use of TENS solely as a last resort modality or by evaluation of only one stimulation mode or electrode array severely hinders its chances of success. TENS efficacy also decreases in proportion to the number of other intervention techniques that have preceeded its use (Wolf et al, 1981).

Stimulation parameters incorporating a high pulse rate (50–100 Hz), narrow pulse width (30–75 µs) and low amplitude (10–30 mA) produce a comfortable tingling sensation or electrical paresthesia without muscle contraction that is consistent with that of conventional TENS. This combination of parameters should selectively activate only large afferent fibers (A alpha and beta) (Linzer & Long, 1974; Burton & Maurer, 1974). Muscle contraction is to be avoided: although dependent upon the electrode array, mild muscle fasciculation is at times hard to eliminate.

On the basis of conventional TENS parameters one should speculate that this mode would be best suited for the control of acute and superficial pain syndromes. Clinical experience, however, has shown that conventional TENS is also frequently beneficial in deep, achy, chronic pain syndromes and therefore remains the most widely used and clinically effective method of TENS.

A decrease in pain perception usually occurs quite rapidly with conventional TENS (1–20 minutes is most common) and upon termination of treatment the duration of relief should at least equal the length of the stimulation period (Linzer & Long, 1974; Burton & Maurer, 1974; Andersson et al, 1977; Andersson & Holmgren, 1978). It is quite common in my clinical experience to see pain relief persist with this mode for one to three hours and occasionally longer. The most important factors that govern the degree and duration of pain relief with any stimulation mode are proper instruction in posture, body mechanics, and activities of daily living (ADL).

Strong low rate

A complete reversal of the stimulation parameters which give rise to the conventional mode, programs the TENS unit to deliver the strong low rate or acupuncture-like mode. Stimulation parameters are consistent with those of invasive electro-acupuncture, but surface electrodes are used in place of subcutaneous needle electrodes (Holmgren 1975; Andersson & Holmgren, 1976).

The strong low rate mode produces intense, rhythmic muscle contractions without the sensation of electrical paresthesia. Depth of stimulus penetration is greater as parameter settings are sufficient to excite high threshold, smaller diameter, slow conducting afferent nerve fibers such as non-myelinated C fibers. Efferent (motor) fibers which require a longer pulse duration for excitation are also activated. Proper programming for this mode requires a low rate (1–4 Hz), wide pulse width (150–250 μs) and amplitude to the highest comfortably tolerable level.

Clinical experience has shown that the strong low rate mode is best suited for deep, achy, chronic pain syndromes. Onset of relief usually does not occur until at least 20–30 minutes of stimulation has elapsed, and at times up to one hour is needed for an adequate evaluation. The duration of post-stimulation analgesia may persist for 2–6 hours or longer (Andersson et al, 1978; Andersson & Holmgren, 1978; Holmgren, 1975; Andersson & Holmgren, 1976; Chapman et al, 1977b; Chapman et al, 1977a; Eriksson & Sjolund, 1976; Eriksson et al, 1979).

Pulse-train

A combination of the parameters inherent in both the conventional and acupuncture-like modes produces what has been termed pulse-train or burst stimulation. High and low pulse rates are utilized simultaneously to deliver a sensation of slow rhythmic pulsing or muscle contractions (dependent upon the total energy per pulse) as well as a background electrical paresthesia. The burst frequency is usually fixed at 2 Hz and high frequency (70–100 Hz) pulses occur within each burst or train (Biostim Inc, 1983; Chapman et al, 1977a; Eriksson et al, 1979; Fox & Melzack, 1976; Mannheimer & Carlsson, 1979).

The pulse-train or burst mode can also be delivered at high or low intensity. Low intensity (without muscle contraction) usage is merely a form of modulating the conventional stimulation mode. Switching from conventional TENS to burst produces a 2 Hz interruption in the steady paresthesia. Patients that do not like the sensation of a constant electrical tingling may prefer to have it interrupted twice each second. The perceived sensation is thus one of electrical paresthesia (from the high frequency pulses per burst) and a rhythmic pulsing twice each second. Clinically, low intensity pulse train (burst) TENS seems to be most effective, as conventional TENS, in acute and/or superficial pain syndromes.

When delivered at high energy levels consistent with that of the strong low rate mode, this form of TENS is known as high intensity pulse-train (burst) stimulation. Stimulation parameters now consist of the same pulse rate but the pulse width and amplitude are increased to a level which produces strong but comfortable muscle contractions (two per second) plus a strong degree of electrical paresthesia. The mixture of both high and low frequency at an energy level sufficient to cause muscle contraction results in an increased recruitment of muscle fibers at less pulse energy than that needed with the strong low rate mode. (Eriksson et al, 1979; Fox & Melzack, 1976).

High intensity pulse-train (burst) TENS seems to be more effective in deep, achy chronic pain syndromes as does the strong low rate mode. The stimulation time required prior to the onset of pain relief and the duration of post-stimulation analgesia with pulse-train (burst) TENS is dependent upon the energy level used and therefore corresponds well to the previously mentioned characteristics of both conventional and strong low rate TENS.

Brief-intense

Brief-intense is the strongest and least tolerable mode, and thus not used as frequently as the other forms. Parameter adjustment for delivery of this mode requires a high rate (100–150 Hz), wide pulse width (150–250 μs) and amplitude to the highest tolerable level that is reasonably comfortable. The resultant sensation is one of a strong and continuous electrical paresthesia that will produce either muscle tetany or nonrhythmic fasciculation depending upon electrode placement. Depth of penetration and stimulus strength is sufficient to excite and recruit the full range of motor and sensory nerve fibers.

Brief-intense TENS gives rise to a rapid onset of analgesia (1–15 minutes), yet the duration of post-stimulation pain relief is quite short. Discomfort usually returns quickly after cessation of stimulation if nociceptive stimuli persist. This is very important to consider when use of this mode is contemplated. It is advisable not to use this mode for periods exceeding 15 minutes as significant ischemia can occur. When pain persists after the use of brief-intense stimulation, a decrease in the total energy per pulse can change the stimulation mode to that of conventional if ongoing pain control is necessary.

The brief-intense mode is primarily employed to obtain quick and profound analgesia which is sufficient to allow for the performance of specific therapeutic procedures such as skin debridement, suture removal, minor dental and podiatric surgical procedures, joint mobilization, transverse friction massage and contract–relax stretching when pain is a hindering factor (Mannheimer & Lampe, 1984a; Mannheimer, 1980; Mannheimer, 1983; Mannheimer & Lampe, 1984b). When TENS is used in this manner, it is recommended that the clinician adhere to the following guidelines:
1. TENS should be initiated 5–15 minutes prior to the onset of the procedure. This should allow for the production of a degree of analgesia sufficient to promote patient tolerance to the therapeutic technique.

2. Stimulation should remain in progress while the technique is being performed.
3. When joint mobilization followed by contract–relax stretching are the desired procedures, active and passive range of motion (ROM) must be assessed before TENS is activated.
4. ROM should not exceed 20 degrees beyond the pretested range in any single treatment session.

These guidelines should eliminate any chance of soft tissue damage. It is important to state at this juncture that TENS allows breakthrough pain to occur. Since the patient is awake (not anesthetized), if pain becomes too unbearable the clinician should be told. Brief-intense TENS obviously does not eliminate all the discomfort of the therapeutic procedure. However, if pain is the one factor that prevents the procedure from being performed at all and TENS can provide at least a 25% decrease in discomfort, then the patient should be able to tolerate some treatment as compared to none at all. I have used brief-intense TENS quite successfully in this manner to rehabilitate patients with functional deficits from adhesive capsulitis (Mannheimer, 1980; Mannheimer, 1983; Mannheimer & Lampe, 1984b). Electrode placement techniques with the brief-intense mode differ in regard to specific therapeutic procedures which are discussed in the electrode placement section.

Brief-intense TENS has also been used to initially break through deep persistent pain in patients with pancreatitis after which management could be achieved by the conventional mode (Roberts, 1978).

Modulation

Modulation of one or more stimulus parameters is the most recent addition to the methods by which TENS can be delivered. Oscillation of pulse rate and/or pulse energy parameters are the most common forms of modulation presently available in newer models manufactured by various companies. The degree of parameter modulation is usually within a range of 40–100%, plus or minus, from the pre-set level. A continuous oscillation occurs within a time factor of $\frac{1}{2}$ to $1\frac{1}{2}$ seconds (dependent upon the manufacturer). Therefore, the number of pulses per second and/or the strength of each pulse shifts back and forth between the pre-set parameter level and the percentage of modulation. A review of the literature relative to the different stimulation modes and a complete listing of their specific characteristics is available (Mannheimer & Lampe, 1984b).

Modulation thus provides for variations in the depth of penetration and recruitment of high and low threshold nerve fibers. The value of modulation is threefold:
1. To increase comfort to irritating but effective stimulation.
2. To increase tolerance to the stronger stimulation modes (strong low rate, and brief-intense).
3. To decrease accommodation to mild continuous stimuli (conventional mode).

Many patients equate the sensation produced by modulation to that of a massage. Factors such as stimulation time prior to the onset of pain relief and its post-stimulation duration are dependent upon the primary mode that is being modulated.

Clinical experience has shown that it is not possible to distinctly categorize each stimulation mode with a list of pain syndromes for which it is best suited. There is no single stimulation mode that is equally effective for all pain syndromes. The mode with the widest range of effectiveness, however, is conventional and thus it should be the first one to be evaluated with any patient or pain syndrome.

Table 4.1 The stimulation modes: Adjustment guidelines

STEP I	STEP II	STEP III	STEP IV	
Mode	Pulse rate	Pulse width	Amplitude	Re-adjustment
Conventional	Pre-set within 50–100 Hz	Pre-set within 40–75 μs	Slowly activate one channel at a time and increase until a smooth comfortable electrical paresthesia is obtained.	Electrical paresthesia should be perceived throughout the distribution of the pain. Increasing the pulse width can result in a spread of paresthesia, comfort can be increased and accommodation minimized by modualtion or burst features.
Strong low rate (acu-puncture-like)	Pre-set 1–4 Hz	Pre-set 150–200 μs	Slowly activate one channel at a time and increase to highest tolerable level producing rhythmic muscle contractions.	Comfort can be increased by use of modulation.

Table 4.1 (con't)

STEP I	STEP II	STEP III	STEP IV	
Mode	Pulse rate	Pulse width	Amplitude	Re-adjustment
Pulse-train burst)	Pre-set within 70–100 Hz or activate fixed burst settings	Pre-set within 40–75 μs (low intensity) 150–200 μs (High intensity)	Slowly activate one channel at a time and increase to desired level. Paresthesia with rhythmic pulsing (low intensity) Paresthesia with rhythmic muscle contractions (high intensity) should occur.	Increasing pulse width can result in a spread of paresthesia if not perceived throughout distributions of pain.
Brief intense	Pre-set within 100–150 Hz	Pre-set within 150–200 μs	Slowly activate one channel at a time to highest tolerable level of paresthesia. Non-rhythmic muscle fasciculations or tetany should occur, in conjunction with paresthesia.	Increase amplitude and/or pulse width if sensation decreases. Activation of modulation can increase comfort and tolerance.

Table 4.1 lists the adjustment guidelines in a step-by-step fashion that should be followed to easily program the different stimulation modes. The suggested settings are to be considered as initial adjustment only. Re-adjustment and adaptation to individual patients and pain syndromes is necessary. Pulse width and amplitude settings can be increased or decreased from the given levels as they are dependent upon the depth and distribution of pain, interelectrode distance, number of electrodes per channel, size of the electrodes and skin resistance. A short inter-electrode distance between two electrodes of one channel will not require a large amount of pulse energy to obtain the desired result.

Principles of electrode placement

A thorough discussion of electrode placement techniques must include information pertaining to optimal stimulation sites and the methods by which the electrode channels are arranged. Electrode placement sites and channel arrangements will also depend upon the specific stimulation mode that is to be used.

In order for TENS to be effective, the stimulus must be transmitted into the central nervous system (CNS). The dense innervation of the skin should permit an adequate stimulus to produce sensory input to the CNS. The strength of the stimulus and its efficacy can, however, be enhanced by electrode placement on optimal stimulation sites (OSS). These sites include the spinal column (specifically paraspinally overlying the posterior primary rami), superficial aspects of peripheral nerves, as well as acupuncture, motor and trigger points. Greater specificity can be obtained by choosing sites at which two or more of the aforementioned entities exist simultaneously.

I have previously published articles and charts which have discussed in detail the anatomical relationship of acupuncture motor and trigger points to one another as well as to superficial aspects of peripheral nerves (Mannheimer, 1978; Mannheimer, 1980; Mannheimer & Lampe, 1984d). These specific points and superficial aspects of peripheral nerves represent anatomical areas that can be distinctly located by a knowledge of musculoskeletal and peripheral neuroanatomy. Futhermore, at least one or more specific points are always found to be located overlying superficial aspects of peripheral nerves. Therefore, stimulation sites used for motor and sensory conduction velocity testing are excellent areas for electrode placement. OSS become tender to palpation in the presence of a segmentally related pathology, are frequently located at indurated areas (bordered by bone), may give rise to referred pain upon pressure and manifest a high electrical conductance with a decreased skin resistance in comparison to the surrounding or adjacent skin (Mannheimer, 1978; Mannheimer, 1980; Mannheimer & Lampe, 1984d). The characteristics of OSS allow them to be easily located by finger palpation. Once the pain distribution has been determined, the therapist should palpate for sites of greatest tenderness within this area concentrating at superficial aspects of peripheral nerves coursing through or innervating the involved region. Palpation should also include muscle bellies, musculotendinous junctions and paraspinally between the transverse processes of segmentally related spinal cord segments. Paraspinal tenderness is manifested at erector spinae motor/trigger points which correspond with bladder meridian acupuncture points as well as posterior primary rami (Mannheimer, 1978; Mannheimer, 1980;

Mannheimer & Lampe, 1984d). The location of OSS can also be performed by scanning the painful region with probes that measure skin resistance (Mannheimer, 1980; Mannheimer & Lampe, 1984d).

When OSS have been determined, the clinician must decide how to arrange the electrodes per channel. Channel arrangements and electrode placement sites may differ according to the stimulation mode. When using the conventional mode, electrode placement and channel arrangements must insure that the sensation of electrical paresthesia is perceived by the patient throughout the entire distribution of pain. This requires at the very least one electrode each at the proximal and distal aspects of the pain distribution. An extensive longitudinal area of pain will necessitate two channels with electrodes arranged in a linear or overlapping pattern. A diffuse area of pain at the posterior aspect of the spine may require a crisscross technique. Electrodes of unequal size per channel may be needed to balance the distribution of electrical paresthesia by adjustments in current density at different skin impedence sites. Electrode placement overlying superficial aspects of related peripheral nerves is recommended.

A prime objective of the strong low rate mode is the production of rhythmic muscle contractions. Electrode placement on motor points of the desired muscle or superficial aspects of the mixed peripheral nerve innervating the specific muscles or myotome will allow for muscle contraction with the least amount of pulse energy. Muscle contractions within the area of pain, especially in the presence of muscle guarding, may not be tolerated by the patient. Effectiveness can still be obtained by electrode placement on motor points of segmentally related myotomes or superficial aspects of innervating peripheral nerves remote from the area of pain. The effectiveness of the strong low rate mode is enhanced by excitation of larger muscle groups.

In the presence of severe low back pain with significant muscle guarding, conventional TENS at the painful region may not be effective. Such a patient will not be able to tolerate the strong low rate mode on the already contracted paraspinal musculature. However, the strong low rate mode may still be effective if electrodes are placed on the legs to produce rhythmic muscle contractions of the gastroc-soleus group. Channel arrangements for this technique would be termed dual channel/bilateral. Electrode placement would be just below the popliteal space and between the medial malleolus and heelcord unilaterally. This array would ensure stimulation of the tibial nerves. These muscles, although remote from the area of pain, are segmentally related via branches of the sciatic nerve which innervate them. Afferent input to the appropiate spinal segments will still occur and may provide activation of pain relief mechanisms. Strong literature support exists for the utilization of segmentally related myotomes Mannheimer & Lampe, 1984b; Mannheimer & Lampe, 1984d; Eriksson et al, 1979; Handwerker et al, 1975; Gunn, 1978).

Electrode placement sites and arrangements with the pulse-train (burst) mode depends upon whether or not high or low intensity is utilized. When high intensity pulse-train stimulation is used, electrode placement sites and channel arrangements will be equivalent to that of the strong low rate mode. The recommendations outlined for the conventional mode holds true when stimulating with low intensity pulse-train TENS.

Brief-intense TENS when applied at superficial aspects of mixed peripheral nerves innervating the area of pain, will produce muscle tetany. This is desired for therapeutic procedures such as skin debridement or suture removal when movement of the involved area is not wanted. When joint mobilization and/or contract–relax stretching is the treatment of choice, electrode placement should not produce muscle tetany as this will hinder joint movement. Electrode arrays for these procedures should produce nonrhythmic muscle fasciculation, and therefore are optimally arranged in a surround or criss-cross fashion at the area of pain and not specifically on superficial peripheral nerve sites. For optimal effectiveness, with the least amount of stimulus strength, electrode placement with the brief-intense mode should be as close to the area of pain as possible.

It is beyond the scope of this chapter to engage in a complete discourse relative to electrode placement techniques and stimulation sites. Several anatomical relationships and physiological processes will be mentioned as they pertain to electrode placement for specific pain syndromes and areas of the body.

Head and face

Electrical stimulation is not tolerated well on the head or face, yet may be required to obtain adequate pain control in the presence of headaches, trigeminal neuralgia, temporomandibular joint syndrome (TMJ) and dental pain. The initial application of TENS in this area should begin at the suboccipital fossa, where stimulation of the occipital nerves as well as the spinal tract of the trigeminal nerve can be accomplished without facial stimulation. Regardless of the specific pain syndromes involving the face or head, a single channel of two electrodes placed in the depression between the cranial attachment of the sternocleidomastoid and upper trapezius muscles should represent the first choice. Bilateral stimulation is recommended, even in the presence of unilateral pain (Mannheimer & Lampe, 1984b; Mannheimer, 1978; Mannheimer, 1980; Mannheimer & Lampe, 1984d).

The spinal tract of the trigeminal nerve has synaptic connections with the upper cervical spinal cord at the C2–C4 level (Elvidge & Li, 1950; Kerr, 1963; Gobel, 1976; Edmeads, 1978). Therefore, suboccipital stimulation may be able to produce pain relief at any facial or cranial region. Electrode placement at the dorsal web space of the hand can also be an effective remote stimulation site to use for control of facial and head pain. Segmental innervation of the dorsal web space is C5–T1 and thus is not considered to be related to the spinal tract of the trigeminal nerve which may extend only as low as the C4 segment. However, upon examination of Penfields' somatomotor and somatosensory cortices one can see an interesting relationship.

Cortical cells which receive input from the thumb and index finger lie adjacent to those of the head and face. The cortical inhibitory surround theory or 'busy cortex' provides a possible explanation for the effectiveness of remote unrelated stimulation sites (Bresler & Froening, 1976; Liao, 1978; Bull, 1973). Significant excitation of a specific cortical region may result in inhibition and decreased sensitivity of an adjacent or surrounding cortical region. Thus, dorsal web space stimulation may cause an increase in the excitation threshold of the cortical cells representative of the face and head. Well-known acupuncture points exist at the sub-occipital fossa (GB20) and dorsal web space (L14) (Mannheimer, 1980).

Electrode placement techniques incorporating both the sub-occipital fossa and dorsal web space can also be evaluated prior to stimulation on the head and face (Mannheimer & Lampe, 1984b; Mannheimer & Lampe, 1984d). Sub-occipital stimulation should not produce muscle guarding, nor promote reflex vasodilation. Thus the conventional mode is recommended. Dorsal web space stimulation can be accomplished with any mode other than brief-intense as long as the patient does not suffer from migraine headaches. Kaada has shown that the pulse-train mode when applied at the dorsal web space in patients with Raynaud's disease produced a 7–10 °C increase in skin temperature and concomitant pain relief, but also resulted in migraine-type headaches in three of four patients (Kaada, 1982).

When stimulation at sites other then the face and head fails to produce satisfactory relief, electrode placement on the head or face may be necessary. This should first be tried with only one electrode at the appropriate area of pain and the other either at the suboccipital fossa or dorsal web space. A small facial electrode and larger sub-occipital or dorsal web space electrode will minimize overflow of stimulation to other facial sites. Low intensity stimulation is necessary in this area and use of a device called the 'Pain Suppressor' which does not exceed 4 mA in amplitude but mediates a pulse rate of approximately 15 000 Hz with a 15 Hz burst, is recommended as an initial application (Mannheimer & Lampe, 1984d). Transcranial stimulation is suggested by the manufacturer (Shealy et al, 1979; Pain Suppression Labs; Markovich, 1977).

Although there is literature support for the efficacy of TENS in trigeminal neuralgia, TMJ and dental pain, reports relating to the use of TENS for headaches are sparse and purely anecdotal (Mannheimer & Lampe, 1984d; Chapman et al 1977a; Markovich, 1977; Mumford, 1976; Appenzeller & Atkinson, 1976; Hag, 1982). The use of TENS in the management of headaches should be purely adjunctive to a comprehensive approach which first determines the specific type of headache and initiates treatment that may consist of biofeedback, relaxation training, postural correction and instruction in proper body mechanics as well as manual techniques for joint and soft tissue dysfunction. Many times such definitive treatment can eliminate the causative factor and dependency upon symptomatic modalities can be negated (Mannheimer & Lampe, 1984d; Sinclair, 1981; Mannheimer & Lampe, 1984e).

Post-operative TENS

The use of TENS post-operatively falls into the category of acute pain management. Hymes has done the pioneering work in the use of TENS after surgery and established its efficacy in a wide variety of thoracic surgical procedures (Hymes, 1984b; Hymes et al, 1975). Post-operative pain control with TENS has also shown a concomitant decrease in the incidence of ileus and atelectasis.

Post-operative TENS is easy to perform once a program has been initiated. The operative site is usually known and electrode placement arrangements are commonly medial and lateral to the incision site. When a second surgical site is present, as in the case of bone taken from a donor site, a dual channel unit will be needed. A dual channel arrangement is also necessary when one pair of electrodes is placed overlying the ascending and descending colon to prevent the development of ileus and the other pair used for pain control at the operative site. Recommended stimulation parameters for post-operative pain control consist of a pulse rate between 50–100 Hz, pulse width of at least 100–200 μs and amplitude to a comfortable level of electrical paresthesia. When an extensive distribution of pain exists, pulse width and amplitude may have to be increased. Parameter modulation can increase tolerance to higher levels of stimulation.

The effectiveness of post-operative TENS has been established for many types of surgery (Ticho et al, 1980; Hymes, 1984b; Hymes et al, 1975; Stabile & Malloy, 1978; Alm et al, 1979; Schuster & Infante, 1980; Harrie, 1979). However, its efficacy is significantly diminished when used with drug-experienced as opposed to drug-naive patients (Solomon et al, 1980). Guidelines for the development and management of a post-operative TENS program are available.

Mode of action

There is no singular explanation for the physiological effects produced by TENS. Each specific stimulation mode may have different sites of action and thus can be explained by more than one theory. The gate control theory has already been mentioned as a plausible explanation for the physiological effects of conventional TENS (Melzack & Wall, 1965; Wolf, 1984). The cortical inhibitory surround theory may be one hypothesis for the action of high frequency TENS, thus explaining some effects of the conventional, pulse-train and the brief-intense modes (Bresler & Froening, 1976; Liao, 1978; Bull, 1973).

Another likely explanation for the effects of high frequency stimulation is simply counter-irritation. Gammon and Starr determined that counter-irritation was most effective when applied at the locus of pain with a pulse rate of 50–60 Hz (Gammon & Starr, 1941)

The stimulation modes that produce strong rhythmic contractions have been shown to promote a release of neurohumeral substances known as enkephalins and endorphins (Andersson, 1979; Eriksson & Sjolund, 1976; Ericksson et al, 1979; Sjolund et al, 1977; Sjolund & Ericksson, 1979; Sjolund & Ericksson, 1976;

Abram et al, 1981). Stimulation requirements, other than strong muscle contractions (high pulse width and amplitude), to produce neurohumoral liberation include a low pulse rate (1–4 Hz) and long induction period of at least 20–30 minutes. Naloxone reversiblity (a return of pain after relief from electrical stimulation upon naloxone administration) has been the criteria used to determine if an endorphin release took place.

Conventional TENS parameters have not shown reversability via naloxone administration (Sjolund & Ericksson, 1979; Sjolund & Ericksson, 1976; Abram et al, 1981). Naloxone is a morphine antagonist available in different strengths and formulations which may effect only selective brainstem sites (Abram et al, 1981; Bausbaum & Fields, 1978; Buchsbaum et al, 1977). There have not been enough definitive studies to strongly support the view that a neurohumoral liberation occurs from strong low rate and high intensity pulse-train TENS. The CSF endorphin level has, however, been elevated by strong low rate TENS (Sjolund et al, 1977).

The best explanation for production of quick analgesia with brief-intense TENS is a conduction block (Ignelzi & Nyquist, 1976; Ignelzi & Nyquist, 1979) The conduction block may be anodal, chemical or ischemic (Mannheimer & Lampe, 1984f). All modes obviously have some effect at the segmental level related to the afferent input that they produce. The stronger modes also have a proposed supraspinal action that does not occur immediately, but possibly produces a summation mechanism. This summation mechanism involves various brainstem structures as well as the pituitary gland and may result in the initiation of neurohumeral liberation which can inhibit the release of substance P, a neurotransmitter needed to promote propagation of afferent nociceptive stimuli (Mannheimer & Lampe, 1984f). A complete discussion of theoretical possibilities relative to TENS, including the complex relationship of serotonin and endogenous opioid peptides, is available (Wolf, 1984; Mannheimer & Lampe, 1984f).

EXAMPLES OF USES OF TENS

Cervical spine

TENS is an excellent adjunctive modality in the comprehensive rehabilitation of patients with acute or chronic cervical spine dysfunction. Nordemar and Thorner found TENS to be very helpful in the management of patients with acute cervical strains (Nordemar

& Thorner, 1981). In my clinical practice, many patients with whiplash injuries benefit from home use of TENS, while out-patient treatment consisting of techniques to restore function, eliminate muscle guarding, remove irritation and eliminate pain is performed. Patients with chronic cervical problems and/or cervical radiculitis also can obtain pain relief with TENS (Mannheimer & Lampe, 1984d).

The conventional stimulation mode with a criss-cross electrode array is recommended for patients with bilateral cervical spine pain from the occipital to the cervical-thoracic junctions or below. When pain is referred from the neck to the upper extremity, a linear current flow with or without the overlapping of stimulation channels is the technique of choice (Mannheimer & Lampe, 1984b; Mannheimer & Lampe, 1984d). Case study No. 1 discusses the adjunctive use of TENS for a patient with occipital neuralgia and headaches. The evaluations, treatment goals and plans for each of the following case studies are taken directly from the patient's charts.

Case study 1

Evaluation. A 64-year-old female referred for treatment on 9/13/83 with a diagnosis of cervical osteoarthritis. History dates to one day in July when she awoke with a 'stiff neck'. She saw her physician who recommended traction at home (18 lb, for 30 minutes, 4×/day). She obtained relief only when the traction was used, but this persisted for a short time after traction. Significant cervical hypomobility existed and she was subsequently hospitalized for 17 days in traction (3 lb) and received treatment solely of TENS and moist heat in the hospital physical therapy department. She was discharged with a Philadelphia collar which she was wearing almost 24 hours per day for the past 2–3 weeks.

The patient complained of periodic sharp pain that was subsequently replaced by an ache. Pain was primarily in the sub-occipital region bilaterally and across the upper trapezius muscles. She also complained of right ear pain, occipital-vertex headaches and left ulnar paresthesia into the 4th and 5th fingers. Paresthesia was present only since the recent hospitalization. Pain was aggravated by combing her hair, coughing, emotional upsets and active movement of the neck. Pain also occurred at night and she slept sidelying on a flat pillow.

Structually there was a significant forward head, round shoulder posture with a Dowager's hump. Active ROM of the cervical spine was severely limited in all directions as follows: forward bending by 50%, backward bending by 80%, bilateral rotation and side-bending by 75% and 85% respectively. There was soft tissue restriction, and pain occurred at end range in all directions. Passive ROM testing revealed similar limitations. Active ROM of the shoulders was within normal limits (WNL).

Strength of the C1–T1 myotomes revealed weakness of the left abductor digiti quinti and first dorsal interosseous which also demonstrated some atrophy. Palpation revealed tenderness of the splenius capitus and upper trapezius muscles bilaterally (L>R). There was some visible muscle guarding at the left paraspinal region. Posterior/anterior (P/A) glides and lateral oscillation of the cervial vertebrae could not be adequately tested as the patient could not assume a prone position. X-ray report stated the presence of neural foraminal encroachment at C3–4 and C4–5 plus narrowing at the C4–5 level with degenerative arthritis.

Goals. Decrease pain, increase function, teach prophylaxis.

Treatment plan. High voltage galvanic stimulation followed by ultrasound, gentle joint mobilization and soft tissue stretching techniques, manual and mechanical (intermittent) traction plus instruction in a home exercise program and proper cervical spine mechanics as well as gradual weaning from the cervical collar. Treatment to be given 3×/week.

This patient had received a TENS unit while in the hospital for home use upon discharge. She, however, was not obtaining satisfactory pain relief with it as electrical paresthesia was not being perceived throughout the entire area of pain. She was using four electrodes at the appropriate stimulation sites (sub-occipital and paraspinal at the cervical-thoracic junction) but channel arrangements were in a longitudinal fashion on each side of the spine.

Figure 4.1 illustrates the electrode placement sites and restructuring of the stimulation channels to that of a criss-cross array. Current flow was thus across the cervical spine producing a greater perception of the electrical paresthesia at the locus of pain. The conventional stimulation mode was used and the patient instructed to place the electrodes on in the A.M and use the unit on an as-needed basis for periods of 20–30 minutes throughout the day.

Progress note. On 10/3/83 the patient was able to go without the cervical collar for the major part of the day, but would develop discomfort if she performed housecleaning or activities requiring forward bending of the head. Pain had decreased in intensity by

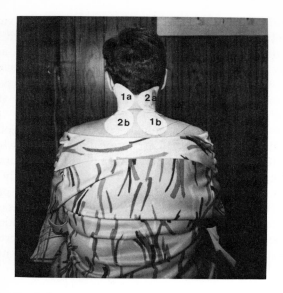

Fig. 4.1 Dx: Cervical osteoarthritis and occipital neuralgia
Electrode placement technique: Criss-cross, dual channel
Electrode placement sites: 1a/2a Sub-occipital 2a/2b, paraspinal at cervical-thoracic junction.
TENS mode: Conventional
Electrodes: Carbon-silicone
TENS unit: Dynex
Rationale: Provides for electrical paresthesia throughout distribution of pain.

50% and occurred periodically. The TENS unit provided at least 75% pain relief when needed and she stopped taking pain medications which had upset her stomach. Active range of motion (ROM) of the cervical spine demonstrated increases in all directions and was now limited by only 15% in forward bending and 50% in bilateral rotation and sidebending as well as backward bending. She was now able to comb her hair much more easily. Treatments were reduced to 2×/week.

Progress note. On 10/24/83 painful episodes continued to decrease in frequency and she was no longer in need of the TENS unit which she was renting from a distributor. Active ROM of the cervical spine had, however, not increased beyond the ranges noted in the previous report. The left ulnar paresthesia remained unchanged and electromyographic studies were suggested. The TENS unit was returned to the distributor and pain relief when needed was being obtained in the form of a home traction unit and ice packs.

Progress note. On 11/14/83 painful episodes were very infrequent and the intensity of pain very low. She, however, complained of bilateral ankle and knee pain which was severe enough to hinder ambulation. The right medial malleolus and left lateral malleolus were red, warm, and edematous. These areas had now replaced the cervical spine pain as her prime concern. This was immediately brought to the attention of the referring physician who subsequently admitted her to the hospital for further evaluation. Treatments were discontinued at this time with increased cervical active ROM noted. Limitations had decreased to 5% in forward bending, 40% in backward bending and sidebending bilaterally, 25% in right rotation and 35% in left rotation.

Upper extremity pain

TENS is an extremely valuable adjunctive pain control modality for intrinsic joint pain, peripheral nerve injuries, amputations, and reflex sympathetic dystrophy (Mannheimer & Lampe, 1984d; Cauthen & Renner, 1975; Stilz et al, 1977; Parry, 1981). Adequate pain control can be obtained by the use of TENS at home to allow for exercise and ROM as well as in the clinic to allow for treatment to be performed. Case study No. 2 highlights the extensive use of TENS for a patient who sustained a traumatic amputation of the distal phalanx of the middle finger.

Case study 2

Evaluation. The patient is a 50-year-old female referred on 7/13/82 for rehabilitation to the right hand. She sustained a traumatic amputation of the distal phalanx of the right middle finger from a machine accident while at work on 3/23/81. Surgical revision was performed on 5/26/81. Post-operatively, she suffered from headaches, right upper extremity (RUE) pain, paresthesia, hyperesthesia of the hand (primarily of the distal end of the amputated finger) which was colder than the adjacent fingers and had a distal sensory deficit. Hand dynamometer readings of 18 kg on the left and 9 kg on the right for grip were obtained.

The finger was hypersensitive to gentle touch and she was unable to tolerate whirlpool due to vibrating irritation. She complained of periodic edema and 'drawing' of the amputated finger along with phantom pain. She returned to work in September of 1981 but could not continue due to increased RUE discomfort. The patient had become depressed and was under care of a psychiatrist.

Active ROM of the right shoulder, elbow and wrist was within normal limits (WNL). Active ROM of the third metacarpal-phalangeal joint (MCP) was WNL but flexion of the proximal inter-phalangeal joint (PIP) was limited to 60 degrees, 75 degrees passively. Active ROM of the cervical spine was limited by 25% in rotation and sidebending bilaterally as well as backward bending.

Goals. Decrease pain and hyperesthesia, increase function.

Treatment plan. Evaluation with TENS for pain control, whirl-pool with high voltage galvanic stimulation followed by ultrasound, joint mobilization and therapeutic exercise as well as instruction in a home exercise program.

The results of the TENS evaluation revealed that five electrodes were needed to obtain adequate pain control (Fig. 4.2). The conventional stimulation mode was used. The patient was only able to perform the home exercise program adequately with simul-taneous use of the TENS unit. Without use of TENS she states that 'the finger feels stiff making it difficult to bend, and pain in the RUE occurs.' TENS also controlled the finger hyperesthesia which allowed for the performance of joint mobilization and manual resis-tive exercise. The patient obtained a TENS unit for home use on rental from a distributor.

Progress note. On 7/29/82 the patient was using the TENS unit daily turning it on about 4×/day for 20 minute periods during which she would exercise.

Progress note. On 9/22/82 the patient was able to make a complete fist and active PIP flexion was measured to 80 degrees. RUE, cervical spine, phantom finger pain and hyperesthesia continued. Purchase of the TENS unit was recommended and agreed upon by the referring physician.

Progress notes. On 11/11/82 pain control still was only possible with TENS. Attempts at various desensitization techniques showed no progress and on 11/17/82 she underwent a second surgical procedure for removal of neuroma formation at the distal end of the amputated finger. She now reported much less pain but had total sensory loss on the volar surface from the PIP crease to the end of the stump. Sensation, however, was intact at the medial, lateral and dorsal surfaces. She reported a vibratory sensation and burning on the dorsum of the finger as well as the palmar surface of the hand whenever she reached for something.

Active ROM had decreased to 50 degrees at the PIP joint and

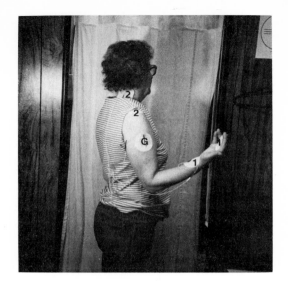

Fig. 4.2 Dx: Reflex sympathetic dystrophy, hyperesthesia and phantom pain following traumatic amputation of distal phalanx of middle finger.
  Electrode placement technique: Linear pathway
  Electrode placement sites: G, common positive at deltoid insertion. Negative electrodes of channel two at right cervical spine and musculotendinous junction of supraspinatus. Negative electrodes of channel one at volar surface of wrist and wrapped around finger proximal to end of stump.
  TENS mode: Conventional
  Electrodes: Carbon-silicone and 'y' adaptors
  TENS unit: Biostim system 10
  Rationale: Electrical parasthesia from the positive electrode to the shoulder and neck and to the forearm and hand to provide pain control throughout whole distribution of pain.

grip strength to 4.5 kg. Between 12/15/82 and 2/2/83 ROM and strength gradually increased, but discomfort of the amputated finger increased. The patient reported pain intensification upon movement which was controlled by TENS. Pain referral to the shoulder and cervical spine increased and active ROM began to decrease. She underwent another surgical revision on 2/23/83 after which she complained of increased pain in the entire RUE and right cervical spine with evidence of causalgia and an apparent reflex sympathetic dystrophy. Treatment in the form of gentle mobilization techniques to the right shoulder and cervical spine was initiated along with intermittent mechanical cervical traction. The patient also obtained a home traction unit as this gave her good relief of cervical discomfort.

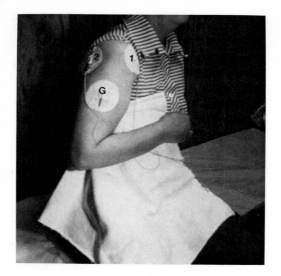

Fig. 4.3 Dx. Reflex sympathetic dystrophy, hyperesthesia and phantom pain following traumatic amputation of distal phalanx of middle finger.

Electrode placement technique: 'V' shaped pathway (3 electrodes)

Electrode placement sites: G, common positive electrode at deltoid insertion. Negative electrode of channel one in depression below acromion anterially; negative electrode of channel two in depression below acromion posterially.

TENS mode: Conventional

Electrodes: Carbon-silicone

TENS unit: Biostim system 10

Rationale: Common positive electrode in series with negative electrodes to produce electrical paresthesia across shoulder.

Note: With a dual (isolated) channel unit a fourth electrode would be placed at the musculotendinous junction (criss-cross technique).

The increased discomfort necessitated evaluation of electrode placement techniques specifically to obtain pain control at the shoulder and cervical spine depicted in Figures 4.3 and 4.4 respectively.

The patient continued to regress and on 9/22/83 she reported that she needed to sleep with the TENS unit on. Relaxation training was initiated. She has since burned the distal volar surface of the amputated finger two times due to sensory loss and a protective splint was fabricated. The patient continued to be very depressed, remained under psychiatric care and continued physical therapy to regain function of the RUE and cervical spine. The TENS unit continued to provide pain relief of at least 75%.

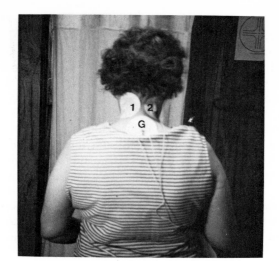

Fig. 4.4 Dx: Reflex sympathetic dystrophy, hyperesthesia and phantom pain following traumatic amputation of distal phalanx of middle finger.
Electrode placement technique: 'V' shaped pathway (3 electrodes)
Electrode placement sites: G, common positive electrode at cervico-thoracic junction midline. Negative electrodes of channel 1 and 2 in sub-occipital fossa.
TENS mode: Conventional
Electrodes: Carbon-silicone
TENS unit: Biostim System 10
Rationale: Arrangement provides for sensation of electrical paresthesia throughout area of pain.

Sensory deprivation pain syndromes

Neuralgia/causalgia and phantom limb pain syndromes fall into the sensory deprivation category. As its name denotes, these pain syndromes result in damage to either large or small afferent nerve fibers thus depriving the CNS of a balanced neural input. Perhaps the best example of sensory deprivation pain syndromes is shingles or herpes zoster (post-herpetic neuralgia).

The herpes zoster virus has an affinity for the myelin sheath and thus selectively attacks the large A fibers dampening the natural CNS proprioceptive input. Normal CNS balance is thus disrupted resulting in a decrease of the excitation threshold of the small diameter nociceptive fibers (Mannheimer & Lampe, 1984e; Sjolund et al, 1977; Ignelzi & Nyquist, 1976; Ignelzi & Nyquist, 1979; Mannheimer & Lampe 1984f; Mudge et al, 1979; Nordemar &

Thorner, 1981; Cauthen & Renner, 1975; Stilz et al, 1977; Parry, 1981; Korr, 1978; Melzack & Loeser, 1978).

Case study No. 3 discusses the role of TENS in the pain management of a patient with a severe case of shingles. The efficacy of TENS in various types of sensory deprivation pain syndromes (SDPS) supports its use in these painful conditions (Mannheimer & Lampe, 1984d; Wolf et al, 1981; Loeser et al, 1975; Meyer & Fields, 1972; Nathan & Wall, 1974; Bates & Nathan, 1980; Long & Hagfors, 1975; Law et al, 1980). Further characterization of SDPS includes cutaneous hyperesthesia induced by non-noxious stimulus, severe intractable burning pain and involvement of the autonomic nervous system. Cutaneous hyperesthesia may negate the placement of electrodes at the involved area. When effective sites cannot be obtained on the side of the lesion, contralateral stimulation of the same dermatomes or peripheral nerve is recommended (Mannheimer & Lampe, 1984d; Laitinen, 1976).

Conventional TENS is the stimulation mode of choice with SDPS as it can produce large A fiber input to the dorsal horn of the cord and hopefully provide a balancing effect. Care must be taken to avoid electrode placement over skin lesions where conduction is likely to be impaired.

Case study 3

Evaluation. A 76-year-old man was referred on 12/13/83 for evaluation with TENS as a means of pain control for post-herpetic neuralgia. The onset of pain was about seven weeks before and skin lesions began within the first week. When seen, scab formation had fallen off but the skin rash remained. The patient also developed nausea, an enlarged abdominal area ipsilateral to the lesion and muscle spasms of the abdominal region which occurred every 30 seconds for two hour periods.

Pain was described as a burning and stabbing type with the feeling of a 'hot needle' in his back. Pain was constant during the day and night and the area of involvement extended from the T10–L1 right paraspinal level laterally and anterior to the umbilicus. Pain was aggravated by sitting, lying on his back or stomach and clothing rubbing against the involved skin area. He was unable to sit upright with his back against a chair. Cold applications and tylenol helped him sleep and he took diazepam (Valium) and percodan daily when pain became severe.

Goals. Establish pain control with TENS.

Treatment plan. The patient arrived with a TENS unit which he had been using at home for the past few weeks. He apparently had not been properly instructed in use of the unit nor evaluated for optimal electrode placement arrangements. He was only using one channel of two small electrodes placed proximal and distal to the skin lesions paraspinally. This arrangement only provided for minimal pain relief at the stimulated area and not the extensive distribution of the pain.

Instruction in operation of the stimulator consisted of turning it on until the electrical sensation appeared and then letting accommodation occur without any further parameter adjustment. He thus was using the unit 24 hours per day but at an intensity that did not provide for the sensation of electrical paresthesia. He stated that he had not been obtaining any significant pain relief.

Due to the extensive area of involvement, large rectangular postoperative electrodes were used in an attempt to block a large area

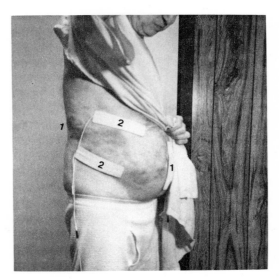

Fig. 4.5 Dx: Herpes zoster (shingles)
 Electrode placement technique: Dual channel criss-cross technique. Channel one electrodes at right paraspinal region (hidden) and to left of midline (anterior) beyond extent of lesions. Channel two electrodes placed superior and inferior to lesions at lateral rib cage.
 TENS mode: Conventional
 Electrodes: Post-operative, karaya by Lec-tec
 TENS unit: 3M Tenzcare
 Rationale: To obtain electrical paresthesia throughout area of pain

of pain. Karaya electrodes were used so that tape would not be required. The initial electrode sites and dual channel array is illustrated in Figure 4.5. This consisted of one electrode pair placed at the right paraspinal region and just to the left of the midline beyond the anterior extent of the lesions. The second pair was placed above and below the lesions at the lateral rib cage. When the unit was activated after re-setting pulse rate and width parameters for the conventional stimulation mode, the patient reported an immediate perception of electrical paresthesia with pain relief throughout the complete distribution of pain beyond that achieved from previous use.

The criss-cross arrangement depicted in Figure 4.6 was chosen as it was assumed that the most intense area of discomfort was the lateral rib cage. The second technique changed the direction of

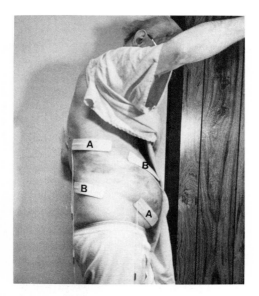

Fig. 4.6 Dx: Herpes Zoster (Shingles)
Electrode placement technique: Dual channel criss-cross technique. Channel A electrodes at superior posterolateral rib cage and inferior anteromedial rib cage. Channel B electrodes at superior anteromedial region to inferior posterolateral rib cage.
TENS mode: Conventional
Electrodes: Post-operative karaya by Lec-tec
TENS unit: 3M Tenzcare
Rationale: An attempt to improve energy flow (electrical paresthesia) across the lateral rib cage.

stimulation to a more distinct 'X' fashion but did not significantly increase benefit.

Upon further questioning, the patient revealed that his most intensive areas of discomfort were at the back and abdomen which thus prompted a rearrangement of the electrodes to two distinctly separate areas as shown in Figure 4.7. This array immediately provided the best pain relief since the interelectrode distance was shortened and independent adjustment of amplitude could be performed as a criss-cross energy flow was not occurring.

Contralateral electrode placement (on the non-involved side) was contemplated. However, this was not attempted as the patient stated that left sidelying was his only comfortable position in which to sleep or rest and he did not want to lie on the electrodes. Instruction was given to keep the electrodes in place 24 hours per day, but to try and turn the stimulation off every hour for at least five to ten minutes or longer if possible. The skin beneath the electrodes was to be checked every six hours. He was told to maintain per-

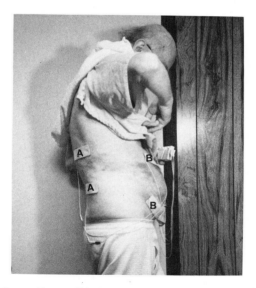

Fig. 4.7 Dx: Herpes Zoster (Shingles)
  Electrode placement technique: Dual channel (isolated).
  Channel A, superior and inferior to lesions at posterior rib cage and spine.
Channel B, superior and inferior to abdominal lesions.
  TENS mode: Conventional
  Electrodes: Post-operative karaya by Lec-tec.
  TENS unit: 3M Tenzcare
  Rationale: Isolate energy at the two most severe regions.

ception of the electrical paresthesia by periodic adjustment of amplitude and/or pulse width at a comfortable level which did not produce muscle contraction.

Follow-up by telephone was performed within a few days as the patient lived a considerable distance away. On 12/20/83 he reported that use of TENS remained continuous with periods of no stimulation not exceeding 30 minutes. He had not had any pain medication since he left the office on 12/13/83. Stimulation was controlling the onset of abdominal muscle spasms which was very helpful to him. Although he continued to experience relatively constant discomfort, the use of TENS was 'now taking the painful edge off' and providing greater relief than anything else (medication or cold applications) that was tried. The percentage of relief was estimated to be about 50% by the patient.

The role of TENS as a means of non-invasive and non-medicinal pain control is perhaps best illustrated in the presence of SDPS. Patients with pain of this intensity and duration which occurs with SDPS can obtain ongoing pain control which usually is not apparent by the use of medication. Furthermore, TENS can accomplish pain control without the side-effects inherent with the use of medication. Proper efficacy, however, can only be obtained in pain syndromes of this type by spending time evaluating the best electrode arrangements. Electrode placement above the level of the lesion is recommended for use with peripheral nerve injuries.

Back and peripheral joint pain

TENS when used properly as an adjunctive technique is also very effective in the control of pain due to arthritic and mechanical dysfunction of the low back and peripheral joints (Mannheimer & Lampe, 1984d; Mannheimer & Carlsson, 1979; Loeser et al, 1975; Mannheimer et al, 1978; Taylor et al, 1981; Kumar & Reford, 1982; Abelson & Langley, 1983).

In fact patients with low back pain constitute the largest pain category in which benefit is obtained from TENS (Walmsley & Flexman, 1979; Paxton, 1980; Gunn & Milbrandt, 1975; Seres & Newman, 1976). It is necessary to reiterate at this point that TENS is not a treatment for low back pain but should merely be used adjunctively for pain control at home while specific therapy to eliminate the cause of pain, correct the dysfunction if possible and prevent recurrence is provided (Mannheimer & Lampe, 1984a; Mannheimer & Lampe, 1984b; Mannheimer & Lampe, 1984c;

Mannheimer & Lampe, 1984e). Case study No. 4 highlights the use
of TENS for a patient with osteoarthritis of the lumbar spine and
left knee.

Case study 4

Evaluation. A 66-year-old female was referred for evaluation with
TENS on 11/7/83. The patient had diagnoses of degenerative
osteoarthritis of the lumbar spine and left knee, compression fractures of L1 and L2 as well as degenerative disc disease. Low back
pain had become a constant ache and was increasing since July. Left
knee pain was periodic and not as severe as the low back.

Back pain was aggravated by ambulation or standing and eased
by sitting upright. Night pain was not a factor, only occurring
slightly when turning. Discomfort was most severe in the a.m. even
though she slept on a firm mattress. Previous treatment in the form

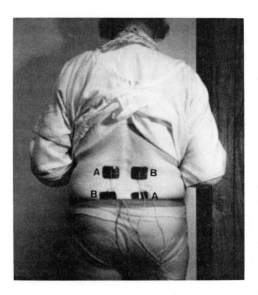

Fig. 4.8 Dx: Degenerative osteoarthritis of lumbar spine and left knee,
compression fractures of L1 & 2
  Electrode placement technique: Dual channel criss-cross. Channel A at left
superior paraspinal area and right inferior paraspinal area. Channel B at right
superior paraspinal area and left inferior paraspinal area.
  TENS mode: Conventional with modulation
  Electrodes: Bioform by Biostim
  TENS unit: Biostim Biomod
  Rationale: Criss-cross electrode array to concentrate energy at center of spine.

of chiropractic kinesiology and the use of medication (motrin and ascriptin) did not provide sufficient pain relief.

The patient ambulated normally. Structurally, there was a significant loss of the lumbar lordosis, rotation of the thoracic spine partially to the right, a forward head and Dowager's hump. Active ROM of the lumbar spine was limited by 75% in backward bending and 50% in sidebending bilaterally with pain at end range. Straight leg raising (SLR) was not limited and did not produce pain. Strength of the L1–S2 myotomes was WNL as was active ROM of the knees.

Posterior/anterior glides and lateral oscillations revealed hypomobility throughout the lumbar spine. Palpation gave rise to local and referred tenderness at the left sciatic notch, popliteal space and superficial aspects of the sural nerve. However, without provocation sciatic pain was not present.

Goals. Obtain pain control with TENS and teach prophylaxis.

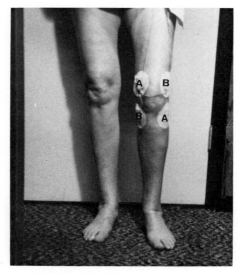

Fig. 4.9 Dx: Degenerative osteoarthritis of lumbar spine and left knee, compression fractures of L1 & L2.

Electrode placement technique: Criss-cross, dual channel

Channel A at right superior to the patella and left by the fibular head. Channel B at left superior to the patella and right inferior with patella

TENS mode: Conventional

Electrodes: Bioform by Biostim

TENS unit: Biostim Biomod

Rationale: Provides a criss-cross current flow across the whole knee.

Treatment plan. Evaluation with TENS determined that satisfactory pain relief was obtained with a dual channel criss-cross technique (Fig. 4.8). The conventional stimulation mode with and without the use of pulse rate and width modulation was preferred for the low back pain. A criss-cross technique about the left knee also provided satisfactory pain relief (Fig. 4.9).

The patient obtained a TENS unit on rental from a dealer on 11/18/83 and was fully instructed in its use. In addition, at this time she was shown how to use one channel at the low back and the other at the left knee to obtain simultaneous pain control at both areas (Fig. 4.10). She was instructed in proper cervical and lumbar spinal mechanics to minimize the degree of pain.

Follow-up telephone conversation on 11/26/83 revealed that the patient was obtaining 75% pain relief which persisted for two or three hours after a 30 minute stimulation period. On the clinic visit of 11/14/83, one month after obtaining the unit for home use, the

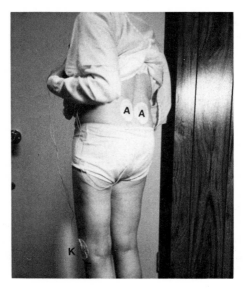

Fig. 4.10 Dx: Degenerative osteoarthritis of lumbar spine and left knee, compression fractures of L1 and 2.
Electrodes placement technique: Dual channel isolated areas. Channel A — bilateral paraspinal, Channel K — bilateral peripheral joint
TENS mode: Conventional
Electrodes: Biostim Bioform
TENS unit: Biostim Biomod
Rationale: Isolated channels to obtain paim controls at two separate areas.

patient decided to purchase it. She was extremely pleased with the benefit obtained and was now getting 90% relief persisting for two to four hour periods after a 30 minute stimulation session. She had been able to eliminate the use of medication and increase her ADL within established guidelines. She was using the unit two or three times per day. The patient was thus discharged and further follow up was done by mail questionnaire.

THE TENS EVALUATION

The successful evaluation of a patient with TENS requires their presence in the clinic at a time of day when pain is most intense and when they are not under the influence of medication (Mannheimer & Lampe, 1984b). The evaluation should be performed in the position which produces pain providing that it is consistent with proper body mechanics. If the patient is unable to assume a proper position due to dysfunction, then the evaluation should proceed in that position and as definitive therapy begins, proper posture should be emphasized.

The conventional stimulation mode should be used for the initial assessment of efficacy. This mode is mild without producing muscle contractions and should provide fast feedback of efficacy. The initial goal is to arrange the electrodes so that perception of the electrical paresthesia is perceived by the patient throughout the complete distribution of pain. Once this has been achieved, the stimulation session should persist for at least 20 minutes. If satisfactory relief is not evident within 20 minutes, the electrodes should be rearranged and tried again. If all possible arrangements using the conventional mode with or without modulation are unsuccessful, further evaluation with another mode should be performed.

My second choice would be the strong low rate or high intensity pulse-train (burst) mode. A proper assessment of the effectiveness of these modes would now require 20–30 minutes at the minimum and possibly up to one hour. Failure to achieve success with any of the aforementioned modes would prompt me to try 5–15 minutes of brief-intense TENS after which pulse width and amplitude parameters would be decreased to the conventional TENS range. Parameter modulation could be used to promote tolerance to brief-intense stimulation.

The prime purpose of the TENS evaluation is to determine the stimulation mode and electrode placement sites and arrangement that provides the patient with the most significant degree of relief that persists the longest with the shortest possible stimulation period. I do not encourage any patient to rent a unit from a dealer unless satisfactory effectiveness is obtained in the clinic. Once this has been determined, the therapist should decide on the specific model and accessories that seem best suited for the patient. Consideration should be given to ease of operation, battery life, lead wire length, electrode size and shape, the transmission medium and form of adherence to the skin. The total package (unit and accessories) should then be ordered from the dealer (a prescription for rental of the device must be obtained) and the patient scheduled for another visit at the time of delivery. As a clinician I do not rent or sell TENS units. This is the domain of the dealer. The dealer should equally respect the domain of the clinician and not perform TENS evaluations.

When the patient is to receive the TENS unit, I first ask him to read the manufacturer's manual in the waiting room and then review the total operation of the device, including electrode maintenance, battery replacement and electrode placement. A complete TENS home instruction form is given to the patient which includes instructions in proper programming of the unit, the desired sensation and length of the treatment period. Electrode placement sites and channel arrangements are drawn on the appropriate page of the instruction form, specific reminders highlighted and the means by which long-term effectiveness will be determined is explained. A complete TENS home instruction form has been developed for patient and clinical use (Lampe & Mannheimer, 1984). If the patient is not being seen for specific treatments, a follow-up appointment is made. If everything is going well, the appointment can be cancelled, but if a problem develops I should be informed. At the very least, I will see the patient one more time just prior to the end of the initial month rental period. A follow-up questionnaire will then be given to the patient to complete in the waiting room or sent by mail if the patient is unable to come to the clinic due to distance (Lampe & Mannheimer, 1984). A determination now needs to be made regarding purchase, continued rental or return of the unit to the dealer if pain has resolved or effectiveness was not satisfactory.

There are numerous factors, separate from proper utilization of the TENS unit, that can interfere with success, enhance it when it is minimal and restore it when it ceases to be effective (Mannheimer & Lampe, 1984f). Perhaps the most important hindering factor is poor body mechanics. Patients with musculoskeletal pain of mechanical origin frequently do not obtain benefit from TENS because they are using the device to obtain pain control while performing improper ADL. The patient with low back pain who leaves the clinic feeling relieved while the TENS unit is functioning and immediately sits in a flexed position in his car will obtain a quick return of pain. Proper instruction by the therapist in the principles of proper body mechanics and postural exercises is of utmost importance to obtain satisfactory relief for a prolonged duration.

The use of specific types of medications or dietary supplements may either hinder, enhance or restore benefit. Valium (diazepam). narcotics and corticosteroids may hinder success while tricyclics and tryptophan may enhance and/or restore efficacy (Mannheimer & Lampe, 1984f; Inversen, 1979; Hosobuchi et al, 1980; Ward et al, 1979).

If the effectiveness of TENS begins to wear off after long-term use, re-evaluation of the patient should be performed to determine if the original quality and distribution of pain has changed. A change in the characteristics of pain may require use of a different stimulation mode and/or electrode arrangement to regain effectiveness.

CONCLUSION

The intent of the chapter has been to provide a complete overview of TENS with emphasis on clinical application. Sections dealing with the stimulation modes, therapeutic applications and the specific adjunctive role of TENS were covered in greater detail than others. TENS is a modality that seems specifically suited for physical therapists as it requires evaluation, hands on application and time to achieve good results. Physical therapists see and treat their patients more frequently than the physician and also have education and training in electrophysiology and electrotherapeutics.

REFERENCES

AAMI Neurosurgery Committee 1981 Proposed Standard for Transcutaneous Electrical Nerve Stimulators. Association for the Advancement of Medical Instrumentation. Arlington

Abelson K, Langley A B 1983 Transcutaneous electrical nerve stimulation in rheumatoid arthritis. New Zealand Medical Journal 96:156

Abram S E, Reynolds A C, Cusick J F 1981 Failure of naloxone to reverse analgesia from transcutaneous electrical stimulation in patients with chronic pain. Anesthesia and Analgesia (Cleve) 60:81

Alm W A, Gold M L, Weil L S 1979 Evaluation of transcutaneous electrical nerve stimulation (TENS) in podiatric surgery. Journal of the American Podiatry Association 69:537

Andersson S A 1979 Pain control by sensory stimulation. In: Bonica J J (ed) Advances in pain research and therapy. Raven Press, New York, p 569

Andersson S A, Holmgren E 1976 Pain threshold effects of peripheral conditioning stimulation. In: Bonica J J, Albe-Fessard D (eds) Advances in pain research and therapy, vol 6, Raven Press, New York, p 761

Andersson S A, Holmgren E 1978 Analgesic effects of peripheral conditioning stimulation III. Effect of high frequency stimulation; segmental mechanisms interacting with pain. Acupuncture and Electro-therapeutics Research 3:23

Andersson S A, Holmgren E, Ross A 1977 Analgesic effects of peripheral conditioning stimulation II. Importance of certain stimulation parameters. Acupuncture and Electro-therapeutics Research 2:237

Appenzeller O, Atkinson R 1976 Transcutaneous nerve stimulation in the treatment of hemicrania and other forms of headache. Minerva Medica 67:2023

Augustinsson L E, Bohlin P, Bundsen P et al 1977 Pain relief during delivery by transcutaneous electrical nerve stimulation. Pain 4:59

Barcalow D R 1919 Electreat relieves pain. Electreat manufacturing company, Peoria

Bates J A V, Nathan P W 1980 Transcutaneous electrical nerve stimulation for chronic pain. Anesthesia 35:817

Bausbaum A I, Fields H L 1978 Endogenous pain control mechanisms: Review and hypothesis. Annals of Neurology 4:451

Biostim Inc 1983 Informative series, Princeton

Bresler D E, Froening R J 1976 Three essential factors in effective acupuncture therapy. American Journal of Chinese Medicine 4:81

Buchsbaum M S, Davis G C, Bunney W E Jr 1977 Naloxone alters pain perception and somatosensory evoked potentials in normal subjects. Nature 270:620

Bull G M 1973 Acupuncture anesthesia. Lancet 2:417

Bundsen P, Ericson K 1982 Pain relief in labor by transcutaneous electrical nerve stimulation: Safety aspects. Acta obstetrica et gynecologica scandinavia 61:1

Burton C, Maurer D D 1974 Pain suppression by transcutaneous electrical stimulation. IEEE Transactions on Biomedical Engineering 21:81

Cauthen J C, Renner E J 1975 Transcutaneous and peripheral nerve stimulation for chronic pain states. Surgical Neurology 4:102

Chapman C R, Chen A C, Bonica J J 1977a Effects of intrasegmental electrical acupuncture on dental pain: evaluation of threshold estimation and sensory decision theory. Pain 3:2131

Chapman C R, Wilson M E, Gehrig J D 1977b Comparative effects of acupuncture on dental pain: evaluation of threshold estimation and sensory decision theory. Pain 3:2131

Edmeads J 1978 Headaches and head pains associated with disease of the cervical spine. Medical Clinics of North America 62:533

Elvidge A R, Li C L 1950 Central protrusion of cervical intervertebral disc involving descending trigeminal tract. Archives Neurology and Psychiatry 63:455

Eriksson M B E, Sjolund B H 1976 Acupuncture-like electro-analgesia in TNS resistant chronic pain. In: Zotterman Y (ed) Sensory functions of the skin. Pergamon Press, Oxford, p 575

Eriksson M B E, Schuller H, Sjolund B H 1978 Letter: Hazard from transcutaneous nerve stimulators: In patients with pacemakers. Lancet 1:1319

Eriksson M B E, Sjolund B H, Neilsen S 1979 Long term results of peripheral conditioning stimulation as analgesic measure in chronic pain. Pain 6:335

Fisher A A 1978 Dermatitis associated with transcutaneous electrical nerve stimulation. Current Contact News 21:24

Fox E J, Melzack R 1976 Transcutaneous electrical stimulation and acupuncture: comparison of treatment of low back pain. Pain 2:141

Furno G S, Tompkins W J 1983 A learning filter for removing noise interference. IEEE Transactions on Biomedical Engineering BME-30:234

Gammon G D, Starr I 1941 Studies on the relief of pain by counter-irritation. Journal of Clinical Investigation 2:13

Gobel S 1976 Principles of organization in the substantia gelatinosa layer of the spinal trigeminal nucleus. In: Bonica J J, Albe-Fessard D (eds) Advances in pain research and therapy. Raven Press, New York p 165

Gunn C C 1978 Transcutaneous neural stimulation: Acupuncture and the current of injury. American Journal of Acupuncture 6:191

Gunn C C, Milbrandt W E 1975 Review of 100 patients with low back sprain treated by surface electrode stimulation of acupuncture points. American Journal of Acupuncture 3:244

Hag K M 1982 Control of head pain in migraine using transcutaneous electrical nerve stimulation. The Practitioner 226:771

Handwerker H B, Iggo A, Zimmerman M 1975 Segmental and supraspinal actions on dorsal horn neurons responding to noxious and non-noxious skin stimuli. Pain 1:147

Harvie K W 1979 A major advance in the control of post-operative knee pain. Orthopedics 2:25

Holmgren E 1975 Increase of pain threshold as a function of conditioning electrical stimulation: An experimental study with application to electroacupuncture for pain suppression. American Journal of Chinese Medicine 3:133

Hosobuchi Y, Lamb S, Bascom D 1980 Trypthophan loading may reverse tolerance to opiate analgesics in humans: A preliminary report. Pain 9:161

Hymes A 1984a A review of the historical area of electricity In: Mannheimer J S, Lampe G N (eds) Clinical transcutaneous electrical nerve stimulation. F A Davis, Philadelphia, p 1

Hymes A 1984b The therapeutic value of postoperative TENS. In: Mannheimer J S, Lampe G N (eds) Clinical transcutaneous electrical nerve stimulation, F A Davis, Philadelphia, p 497

Hymes A C, Yonehiro E G, Raab D E et al 1975 Electrical surface stimulation for treatment and prevention of ileus and atelectasis. Surgical Forum 26: 222–224

Ignelzi R J, Nyquist J K 1976 Direct effect of electrical stimulation on peripheral nerve evoked activity. Implications for pain relief. Journal of Neurosurgery 45:159

Ignelzi R J, Nyquist J K 1979 Excitability changes in peripheral nerve fibers after repetitive electrical stimulation: Implications in pain modulation. Journal of Neurosurgery 51:824

Inversen L L 1979 The chemistry of the brain. Scientific American 241:134

Kaada B 1982 Vasodilation induced by transcutaneous nerve stimulation in peripheral ischemia (Raynaud's) phenomenon and diabetic polyneuropathy. European Heart Journal 3:303

Kerr F W L 1963 Mechanisms, diagnosis and management of some cranial and facial pain syndromes. Surgical Clinics of North America 43:951

Korr I M 1978 Sustained sympathicotonia. In: Korr I M (ed) The neurobiologic mechanisms in manipulative therapy. Plenum Press, New York, p 229

Kumar U N, Redford J B 1982 Transcutaneous nerve stimulation in rheumatoid arthritis. Archives of Physical Medicine and Rehabilitation 63:595

Laitinen L 1976 Placement of electrodes in transcutaneous stimulation for chronic pain. Neuro-chirurgie 22:517

Lampe G N, Mannheimer J S 1984 Postoperative TENS analgesia: Protocol, methods, results and benefit. In: Mannheimer J S, Lampe G N (eds) Clinical transcutaneous electrical nerve stimulation. F A Davis, Philadelphia, p 511

Lampe G N, Mannheimer J S 1984 The patient and TENS. In: Mannheimer J S, Lampe G N (eds) Clinical transcutaneous electrical nerve stimulation. F A Davis, Philadelphia, p 219

Law J D, Swett J, Krisch W M 1980 Retrospective analysis of 22 patients with chronic pain treated by peripheral nerve stimulation. Journal of Neurosurgery 52:482

Liao S J 1978 Recent advances in the understanding of acupuncture. Yale Journal of Biology and Medicine 51:55

Linzer M, Long D M 1974 Transcutaneous neural stimulation for relief of pain. IEEE Transactions on Biomedical Engineering 23:341

Loeser J S, Black R G, Christman A 1975 Relief of pain by transcutaneous stimulation. Journal of Neurosurgery 42:308

Long D M, Hagfors N 1975 Electrical stimulation of the nervous system: The current status of electrical stimulation of the nervous system for relief of pain. Pain 1:109

Long D M, Campbell J N, Gucer G 1979 Transcutaneous electrical stimulation for relief of chronic pain. Advances in Pain Therapy 3:593

Mannheimer J S 1978 Electrode placement for transcutaneous electrical nerve stimulation. Physical Therapy 58:1455

Mannheimer J S 1980 Transcutaneous electrical nerve stimulation for pain modulation during specific therapeutic techniques. Program Abstracts, second general meeting of the American Pain Society 56

Mannheimer J S 1980 Optimal stimulation sites for TENS electrodes. Trenton, Hibbert Co

Mannheimer J S 1983 TENS as an adjunctive technique in hand rehabilitation. APTA Hand Section newsletter

Mannheimer J S 1983 TENS Update: The stimulation modes. Stimulus, Clinical Electrophysiology Section of APTA 8:10

Mannheimer C, Carlsson C A 1979 The analgesic effect of transcutaneous electrical nerve stimulation (TENS) in patients with rheumatoid arthritis. A comparative study of different pulse patterns. Pain 6:329

Mannheimer J S, Lampe G N 1984a Pain and TENS in pain management. In: Mannheimer J S, Lampe G N (eds) Clinical transcutaneous electrical nerve stimulation, F A Davis, Philadelphia, p 7

Mannheimer J S, Lampe G N 1984b Electrode placement techniques. In: Mannheimer J S, Lampe G N (eds) Clinical transcutaneous electrical nerve stimulation. F A Davis, Philadelphia, p 331

Mannheimer J S, Lampe G N 1984c Clinical transcutaneous electrical nerve stimulation. F A Davis, Philadelphia

Mannheimer J S, Lampe G N 1984d Electrode placement sites and their relationships. In: Mannheimer J S, Lampe G N (eds) Clinical transcutaneous electrical nerve stimulation.. F A Davis, Philadelphia, p 249

Mannheimer J S, Lampe G N 1984e Differential evaluation for the determination of TENS effectiveness in specific pain syndromes. In: Mannheimer J S, Lampe G N (eds) Clinical transcutaneous electrical nerve stimulation. F A Davis, Philadelphia, p 63

Mannheimer J S, Lampe G N 1984f Factors that hinder, enhance and restore the effectiveness of TENS: Physiologic and theoretical considerations. In: Mannheimer J S, Lampe G N (eds) Clinical transcutaneous electrical nerve stimulation. F A Davis, Philadelphia, p 529

Mannheimer C, Lund S, Carlsson C A 1978 The effect of transcutaneous electrical nerve stimulation (TENS) on joint pain in patients with rheumatoid arthritis. Scandinavian Journal of Rheumatology 7:13

Markovich S E 1977 Pain in the head: A neurological appraisal. In: Gelb H (ed) Clinical management of head, neck and TMJ pain and dysfunction. W B Saunders, Philadelphia, p 125

Melzack R, Loeser J D 1978 Phantom body pain in paraplegics: Evidence for a central pattern generating mechanism for pain. Pain 4:195

Melzack R, Wall P W 1965 Pain mechanisms: A new theory. Science 150:971

Meyer G A, Fields H C 1972 Causalgia treated by selective large fiber stimulation of the peripheral nerve. Brain 95:163

Mudge A W, Leeman F E, Fishbach G D 1979 Enkephalin inhibits release of substance P from sensory neurons in culture and decreases action potential duration. Proceedings of the National Academy of Sciences of the USA. 76:526

Mumford J M 1976 Relief of orofacial pain by transcutaneous neural stimulation. J Br Endo Soc 9:71

Nathan P W, Wall P D 1974 Treatment of postherpetic neuralgia by prolonged electrical stimulation. British Medical Journal 3:645

Nordemar R, Thorner C 1981 Treatment of acute cervical pain — a comparative study group. Pain 10:93

Pain Suppression Labs, Inc. 559 River Road, Elmwood Park, New Jersey

Parry C B W 1981 Rehabilitation of the hand, 4th edn. Butterworths, London, p 129

Paxton S L 1980 Clinical use of TENS: A survey of physical therapists. Physical Therapy 60:38

Peper A, Grimbergen C A 1983 EEG measurement during electrical stimulation. IEEE Transactions on Biomedical Engineering BME-30:231

Ray C D 1977 New electrical stimulation methods for therapy and rehabilitation. Ortho Review 4:29

Roberts H J 1978 Transcutaneous electrical nerve stimulation in the management of pancreatitis pain. Southern Medical Journal 71:396

Schuster G, Infante M 1980 Pain relief after low back surgery: The efficacy of transcutaneous electrical nerve stimulation. Pain 8: 299–302

Seres J L, Newman R I 1976 Results of treatment of chronic low back pain at the Portland Pain Center. Journal of Neurosurgery 45:32

Shealy C N, Maurer D 1974 Transcutaneous nerve stimulation for control of pain. Surgical Neurology 2:45

Shealy C N, Mortimer J T 1970 Dorsal column electro-analgesia. Journal of Neurosurgery 32:560

Shealy C N, Kwako J L, Hughes S 1979 Effects of transcranial neurostimulation upon mood and serotonin production: A preliminary report. Il Dolore 1:13

Shealy C N, Mortimer J T, Reswick J B 1967 Electrical inhibition of pain by stimulation of the dorsal column: Preliminary clinical reports. Anesthesia and Analgesia (Cleve) 45:489

Sinclair D 1981 Mechanisms of cutaneous sensation. Oxford University Press, Oxford

Sjolund B H, Eriksson M B E 1976 Electro-acupuncture and endogenous morphine. Lancet 2:1035

Sjolund B H, Eriksson M B E 1979 The influence of naloxone on analgesia produced by peripheral conditioning stimulation. Brain Research 173: 295–301

Sjolund B H, Terenius, Eriksson M B E 1977 Increased cerebrospinal fluid levels of endorphin after electroacupuncture. Acta physiologica scandinavia 100:382

Sjolund B H, Terenius L, Ericksson M B E 1977 Increased cerebrospinal fluid levels of endorphin after electro-acupuncture. Acta physiologica scandinavia 100: 382–384

Solomon R A, Viernstein M C, Long D M 1980 Reduction of postoperative pain and narcotic use by transcutaneous electrical nerve stimulation. Surgery 87:142

Stabile M L, Malloy T H 1978 The management of post-operative pain in total joint replacement. Ortho Review 7:121

Stilz R J, Carron H, Sanders D B 1977 Case history number 96: Reflex sympathetic dystrophy in a 6 year old: Successful treatment by transcutaneous nerve stimulation. Anesthesia and Analgesia 56:438

Taub A, Kane K 1975 A history of local analgesia. Pain 1:125
Taylor P, Hallet M, Flaherty L 1981 Treatment of osteo-arthritis of the knee
with transcutaneous electrical stimulation. Pain 11:233
Thorsteinsson G, Stonnington H H, Stillwell G K et al 1978 The placebo effect of
transcutaneous electrical nerve stimulation. Pain 5:31
Ticho U, Olshwang D, Magora F 1980 Relief of pain by subcutaneous electrical
stimulation after ocular surgery. American Journal of Opthalmology 89:803
Walmsley R P, Flexman N E 1979 Transcutaneous nerve stimulation for chronic
low back pain: A pilot study. Physiotherapy Canada 31:245
Ward N G, Bloom V L, Friedel R O 1979 The effectiveness of tricyclic
antidepressants in the treatment of co-existing pain and depression. Pain 7:331
Wolf S L 1984 Neurophysiologic mechanisms in pain modulation: Relevance to
TENS. In: Mannheimer J S, Lampe G N (eds) Clinical transcutaneous
electrical nerve stimulation. F A Davis, Philadelphia, p 41
Wolf S L, Gersh M R, Rao V R 1981 Examination of electrode placement and
stimulation parameters in treating chronic pain with conventional electrical
nerve stimulation (TENS). Pain 11:37

Acupuncture and acupressure

Acupuncture and acupressure are widely accepted as useful modalities with which to treat pain. These methods can be used in general practitioners' offices, physiotherapists' clinics, anaesthesiologists' pain clinics, and in operating theatres. In China this form of treatment has been in use for over five thousand years but Western scepticism, together with China's inaccessibility, prevented its recognition and growth throughout the Western world until the nineteenth and twentieth centuries. Research is now producing scientific data which verify the value of acupuncture, and gradually it is becoming more readily available to the public as a method of treatment. Acupuncture's most widely recognised use is in the treatment of pain but its beneficial effects encompass several other fields. Training and skill in acupuncture and/or acupressure would be a valuable asset to all physiotherapists who treat painful conditions responsive to this form of treatment.

HISTORY

According to an old Chinese fable acupuncture was discovered by a warrior who was wounded by an arrow during battle. When shot by a second arrow he realised that he could no longer feel the pain from the first. It was later deduced that this second arrow had punctured an area which effected his appreciation of pain.

During the Han dynasty (206 BC to 220 AD) acupuncture was performed with a sharp stone—a pien. This pien was used to prick certain parts of the body with resultant relief of pain. Needles of bone and bamboo were later used and eventually, with the discovery of metals, metallic needles came into use.

A comprehensive book was written during the Tsin Dynasty (265 AD to 420), describing 349 basic acupuncture points. In the eleventh century, students were instructed in the art of acupuncture using bronze figures with holes marking the location of points.

The political climate in China during the Ching dynasty (1644 to 1911) discouraged the practice of traditional acupuncture. After the Republic of China was established acupuncture was banned and Western medicine encouraged. In 1949 with the expulsion of Chang Kai-Shek's nationalist government and the take-over of Mao Tse-Tung's communist-based People's Republic, policies were reversed and traditional medicine was again encouraged, this time alongside Western medicine.

During the 1966 cultural revolution all Chinese societies, including medical schools, closed and no communication between the Western and Chinese medical worlds existed. Communication re-started in 1970 after the commencement of a three-year medical course in China. The course included both traditional Chinese and Western methods of treatment. In 1973 the publication of medical journals in China resumed and information was again available to the West. Today acupuncture is used in most countries of the world.

CHINESE PHILOSOPHY

To understand the traditional Eastern acupuncture concept one must have some knowledge of Chinese philosophy. The decisions about which points to use for treatment are based on this philosophy.

Yin and Yang

The Chinese accept a concept of Ch'i or life force. This, they believe, is present throughout the universe. Ch'i consists of two ever changing aspects called yin and yang. Yin and yang are simultaneously complementary and opposite; e.g. male and female, or cold and hot. Everything in nature can be grouped into either yin or yang but, as nothing is absolute, all things yin contain a small amount of yang and vice versa. It is of fundamental importance to maintain the equilibrium between yin and yang. Disease occurs when this state of equilibrium, either within an individual's body or within the universe, becomes imbalanced.

Meridians

The Chinese believe that Ch'i, i.e. yin and yang, flows through the body along channels called meridians. There are twelve of these channels which occur bilaterally, and two central channels. Inter-linking channels also exist between these main meridians. The main channels connect with the viscera and many are named accordingly, e.g. lung meridian of hand-taiyin, kidney meridian of foot-shaoyin. Parts of some of these channels relate closely to nerves.

Acupuncture points

These are approximately seven hundred anatomically described areas, lying along meridians, where stimulation is applied during treatment (The Academy of Traditional Chinese Medicine, 1975). These points have been shown to be areas of decreased skin resistance, and they often correspond to motor or trigger points.

Pulse diagnosis

Pulse diagnosis plays an important part in choosing which meridian or meridians should be used for selection of points for treatment.
   On each wrist, over the radial artery, six pulses can be felt. Each pulse relates to the function of an organ or meridian, and an experienced clinician can, by palpation of these pulses, diagnose an imbalance on a particular meridian. He then selects points along that meridian to treat.

Energic cycles

There are several of these cycles in traditional acupuncture theory, all of which have relevance when selecting points for treatment.
   The most commonly used cycles are called cheng cycle and co cycle. The cycle concept supplies a sequence whereby one organ and/or meridian influences another. The cheng cycle is energising, the co cycle controlling. Having made a pulse diagnosis of, for example, a bladder meridian problem, the clinician may decide to treat points on the bladder meridian. He may instead decide to treat points on the colon meridian or the stomach meridian as these two channels can effect the bladder meridian. In Western medical terms, it can be accepted that these organs are all related and disease of one may effect the other.

Chinese clock

The Chinese have a concept that energy flows through particular organs and meridians in a specific order and at a specific time of

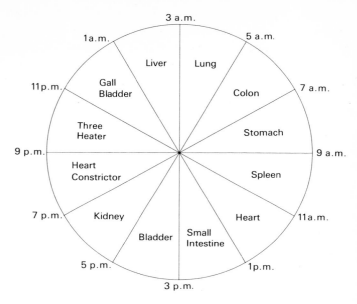

Fig. 5.1 Chinese clock

day or night (Fig. 5.1). Energy is said to 'commence' in the lungs at 3 a.m., and remains at a high level until 5 a.m. when it flows into the colon for two hours, then to the stomach, spleen, heart and throughout the entire body. If the lung meridian is at its peak energy at between 3 a.m. and 5 a.m., it is also at its lowest energy level at between 3 p.m. and 5 p.m. Treatment for a diseased organ or meridian is most beneficial if it can be done during the peak energy time, although in a clinical situation this is not always appropriate.

In Western terms everything in nature is known to be cyclical, so the Chinese clock concept may not be as strange as it first appears.

Five elements

The Chinese group everything, e.g. diseases, temperament, organs, tastes, seasons, climatic conditions, human tissues, etc. into five groups. These groups, or elements as they are referred to in Chinese medicine, are fire, earth, metal, water and wood (Fig. 5.2). The twelve major meridians fit into these groups in pairs, e.g. the spleen and stomach meridians are in the earth element, bladder and kidney

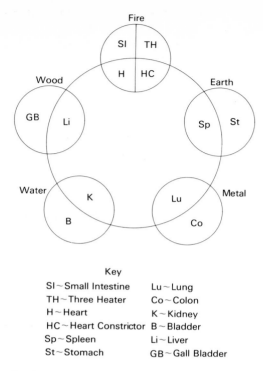

Key

SI ~ Small Intestine   Lu ~ Lung
TH ~ Three Heater   Co ~ Colon
H ~ Heart   K ~ Kidney
HC ~ Heart Constrictor   B ~ Bladder
Sp ~ Spleen   Li ~ Liver
St ~ Stomach   GB ~ Gall Bladder

Fig. 5.2 Five elements

are in the water element, and gall bladder and liver belong to the element wood.

Based on the element grouping, the Chinese see connections between human organs or tissues and many other factors which the Western medically trained clinician would not necessarily recognise, e.g. lung and colon meridians are associated with skin, smell and mucous, while gall bladder and liver meridians are associated with muscles, vision, and tears. This concept influences the choice of meridians and points for treatment.

Rules of acupuncture

The rules of acupuncture allow the clinician to decide which points to use for treatment. Briefly, they are as follows:
a. points in the area of symptoms
b. end points of all the meridians close to the area of symptoms

c. points local to the site of symptoms together with distant points on the same meridian
d. points with recognised special action, e.g. colon 4 for pain, spleen 6 for gynaecological problems
e. key points, which are single points which control more than one meridian
f. points selected based on pulse findings and five element associations
g. associated effect points, which are bladder meridian points with specific action on other organs, e.g. bladder 13 for lung conditions, bladder 21 for stomach conditions
h. use of formulae, which are groups of points that are recognised as being of value in specific symptoms, for example colon 4 and liver 3 for anxiety, stomach 34, 35, and spleen 10 for knee pain
i. points in opposition, i.e. if a particularly strong effect is required use a relevant point on the opposite side of the body to the symptoms
j. points in a line, i.e. a greater effect is produced by stimulating several adjacent points on the same meridian, e.g. for low back pain bladder 22, 23 24 and 25 situated adjacent to the transverse processes of L_2, L_3, L_4, and L_5 respectively are often used.

PRACTICAL TECHNIQUES

Point location

There are several methods of locating points. Initial reference to a chart showing anatomical relationships of the points to be treated is the first step. Felix Mann's *Atlas of Acupuncture*, published by William Heinemann Medical Books Ltd, London (1966) is an excellent chart for this purpose.

Palpation is the next step. Often the points are painful to deep palpation in a normal subject, e.g. spleen 10 at Vastus Medialis motor point. Points which are not normally painful but become so when symptoms are present are usually useful to stimulate. Often points lie in tissue depressions, e.g. colon 7 on the posterior aspect of the forearm and colon 5 in the anatomical snuff box at the wrist. As with all palpation, practice improves one's ability to perceive the relevant information.

Point detectors can be used that resemble pen-like instruments which measure the skin resistance to electric current. The detectors signal when areas of lowered resistance are found. Care is required when selecting such an instrument as some will signal incorrectly when the hand pressure of the operator alters.

Types of stimulation

There are many methods by which acupuncture points can be stimulated, e.g. needle insertion, pressure, heat, electric current, vibration, ultrasound, laser. All of these techniques are useful, and generally the greater the stimulation the greater the response.

Acupuncture

For a physiotherapist to perform this treatment safely and effectively it is essential for her to have had specialised training in needling technique. There are dangers of infection including hepatitis contamination, and of puncturing vital organs, especially the lungs. Individual differences in the surface markings of the lungs and other organs cannot always be recognised.

Needles are usually made of stainless steel although silver and gold are available and may be more appropriate in some conditions. Needles vary in length and diameter, but the most commonly used are $\frac{1}{2}$ to 2 in. long with a diameter of 28 to 32 gauge. Press needles are also available for auricular acupuncture. These are $\frac{1}{16}$ inch in length. Sterilization of all needles is essential.

When a needle is inserted into an acupuncture point the operator must quickly rotate it for a few seconds until the patient describes a sensation of heaviness, or tingling, or numbness in the area. This is known in Chinese as Teh Ch'i, i.e. activating the energy flow. The needle should be withdrawn after one to twenty minutes depending on the sensitivity of the patient and the desired effect. It may be rotated manually or electrically for all, part, or none of this time, again depending on the degree of stimulation required. I have used electroacupuncture when brief manual rotation with the needle in situ for fifteen minutes has not achieved the desired effect.

Electroacupuncture

Electroacupuncture is the attachment of an electrode to the handle of the acupuncture needle. Several needles may be simultaneously attached and stimulated. Many types of machines are available with low and high frequency variations. Omura (1978) notes that for the same pulse wave-form, the higher the frequency, the shorter the time it takes to induce the maximum analgesic effect, but the duration of the effect is reduced.

Moxibustion

This is a method of applying heat to an acupuncture point. It may be applied to a needle in situ resulting in heat penetration to the depth of the needle, or, when needles are not being used, it may be applied superficially to the skin area overlying the point. The traditional method of applying heat is by use of moxa. This is a herb, Artemis Vulgaris, and is sold either loosely in bags or packed in a cigar-shaped form.

To attach moxa to a needle one places a small amount around the needle handle while the needle is in situ. It is then lit and allowed to smolder slowly. This should not cause discomfort, only a sensation of warmth. When needles are not being used, one should light one end of the 'cigar' and hold it perpendicular to the skin over the acupuncture point but not in contact with the body surface. The patient is instructed to inform the operator immediately if the heat becomes intense, at which time the moxa is withdrawn. Heat is applied in this way approximately six or seven times to each point being treated.

Acupressure

This is a means of stimulating acupuncture points without using needles. It is a valuable and easily learned skill. It is particularly popular in Japan where it is called Shiatsu—Shi meaning finger and atsu meaning pressure. The traditional concepts of Shiatsu are exactly the same as those of acupuncture, incorporating energy flow along yin and yang meridian lines and points where this energy can be influenced. These points are the same as those for acupuncture but are called tsubo.

If one has training in acupuncture techniques, one would only use acupressure in certain situations, such as:
a. in patients with pain who were unwilling to have, or anxious about being given acupuncture
b. in treatment of children who may be frightened by a needle
c. teaching patients self-treatment
d. in any patient whom the operator suspects may be supersensitive to acupuncture (Takeshige, 1980)
e. severely debilitated patients
f. if needles were not available.

Pressure may be applied with a finger or thumb, or any blunt instrument. Many techniques can be used, e.g. massage in a circular motion for between three and five minutes, pressing inwards towards the centre of the body for approximately 10 seconds repeated three times, or vibrating the point with finger tip pressure. Like acupuncture, the value of acupressure is not limited to the treatment of painful conditions but is a useful tool when pain occurs.

Auricular acupuncture

This is acupuncture to the outer ear where particular areas can be used to treat conditions of particular parts of the body. Acupressure can also be used if needles are inappropriate.

Auricular acupuncture is a newer concept than torso or limb acupuncture but the connection between the ear and sciatic pain was referred to in writings by Hippocrates.

The relationship between various parts of the body and areas on the ear are shown in Figure 5.3. Needles placed in these areas can result in pain relief in the affected part. Nogier (1972) describes these ear correspondences as being 0.2 mm diameter in width, and their placement is somewhat variable in different patients. Points

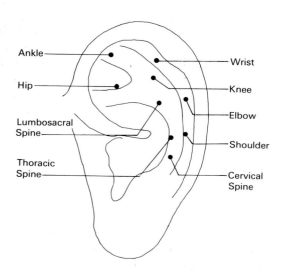

Fig. 5.3 Approximate positions of body areas on the ear

are located by palpation, initially by hand and then with a spring-loaded feeler to detect the precise point, or by electric stimulator (Cho & Cho, 1978). The correct point is usually painful when symptoms of the related part are present. The point may also be anaesthetic to hot or cold palpation.

The auricular cardiac reflex (ACR) may also be used to detect ear points. This reflex, discovered by Nogier, results in an alteration of pulse speed or strength, felt by the clinician at the radial artery, when the painful point on the ear corresponding to the area of the patient's symptoms is stimulated with a blunt instrument.

The selection of needles is important in auricular acupuncture. If the patient's condition is aggravated by movement choose gold needles, if aggravated by rest choose silver, and if there is mixed aggravation use steel. The precise change recorded in ACR will indicate which metal is appropriate (Nogier, 1972).

Auricular acupressure

Acupressure is also very useful in auriculotherapy. Nogier advises the use of a glass rod with a smooth, curved agate tip with which to do 'micro massage' to the appropriate painful ear point. He notes that initially the response is that of increased local ear sensitivity followed by a decrease in both the ear pain and the pain of the area of original symptoms (Nogier, 1972). The pressure applied is incorporated with friction over an area not exceeding 1 cm in length. Nogier further notes that the direction of the massage is of prime importance, and the operator must massage first in one direction, then in the other and finally perpendicularly. The direction chosen should be the one which causes least local discomfort to the patient. The friction movement should be repeated eight to ten times. As with ear acupuncture, the ear to treat is usually that on the same side of the body as the symptoms.

Auriculotherapy case history

Nogier cites recent trauma as his main indication for use of auriculotherapy, with pain being one of the main symptoms. I have used ear acupuncture in cases when improvement has ceased with other methods. One such case was a patient with periarthritis of his shoulder. His range of movement and pain had improved and then

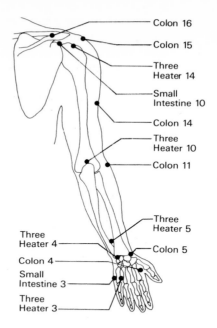

Colon 16
Colon 15
Three Heater 14
Small Intestine 10
Colon 14
Three Heater 10
Colon 11
Three Heater 5
Three Heater 4
Colon 5
Colon 4
Small Intestine 3
Three Heater 3

Fig. 5.4 Some commonly used points on the posterior aspect of the arm.

plateaued with physiotherapy. I then used acupuncture to points on the colon, three heater and small intestine meridians around the shoulder (Fig. 5.4). His range and pain showed further improvement but again plateaued. I added electroacupuncuture with the same result, and finally used electroacupuncture on an appropriate painful point on his ear (Fig. 5.3). This resulted in immediate total loss of pain and marked improvement in range and the patient was able to return to his manual job.

Nogier stresses the fact that in cases of joint symptoms manual therapy is often the first treatment approach, but when symptoms are still present afterwards, then auriculotherapy is appropriate. The majority of his patients come to him with a history of having achieved unsatisfactory relief of symptoms with various therapies. He reports that approximately four treatments are required, spaced several days or several weeks apart depending on the duration of symptoms, i.e. the more chronic the case the greater time lapse between treatments. If auriculotherapy is going to be successful some relief of pain should occur within a minute of the first application of treatment.

TREATMENT

Selection of patients

Patients are selected for acupuncture for a variety of reasons including:

a. referral from therapists when other means of treatment have failed
b. self-selection or when the patient requests acupuncture. These patients have often had a variety of previous treatments with unsatisfactory results
c. as the therapist's first attempt at pain relief
d. where the therapist decides to use acupuncture in conjunction with other therapies.

Groups (a) and (b) above are the most difficult cases but results can be good. In a trial of acupuncture into motor points for chronic low back pain, Gunn et al (1980) report a significantly better response in patients treated with acupuncture plus physiotherapy than in those treated only with physiotherapy.

Group (b) is often the smallest group of patients in Western clinics. In the Orient this is not so as a visit to the Acupuncturist is often the patient's first line of approach.

In a physiotherapy department, group (d) may be the area where acupuncture or acupressure find most use. These therapies may be added to a series of treatments which a patient is undergoing. If a particular mobilization or manipulation is known to have a specific beneficial effect on a patient, then acupuncture may be included beforehand to enhance this effect. I have found acupuncture useful prior to friction massage when the latter had caused too great an intensity of pain.

It is essential that a patient relaxes during acupuncture. If he is overanxious, needling will cause pain and no benefit will result. For this reason acupuncture should not be used on an unwilling patient. Acupressure, instead, can be a very useful therapy in these cases.

Patient examination

The same principles and methods of examination apply whether or not one is considering acupuncture or acupressure as well as standard physiotherapy as a means of treatment. There are, however, a few additions to the examination which are relevant to acupuncture. These are as follows:

a. Past medical health. This area is considered in more detail than for usual physiotherapy assessments, due to the relationship seen between organ function and areas of the body. A special question relating to history of hepatitis is most relevant to acupuncturists. A positive response does not contraindicate treatment as needles may be kept solely for use on one patient. However, hepatitis carriers may not be detected by questioning and for this reason autoclaving of equipment is advisable.

b. Holistic history. This consists of questioning about menstrual, emotional, social, diet, and sleep patterns. In this way the therapist gains a holistic impression of the patient.

c. Pulse diagnosis. This requires training and experience (p. 124)

d. Palpation of associated effect and alarm points. These are specific points which, if tender, may indicate the source of the patient's problem. They are fully described in *An Outline of Chinese Acupuncture*, produced by the Academy of Chinese Medicine, and published in Peking by the Foreign Languages Press (1975), in which they are referred to respectively as Back-shu and Mu-front points. The Back-shu points lie on the bladder meridian on the posterior aspect of the trunk, and the Mu-front points lie on the anterior aspect of the chest and abdomen.

e. Observation and/or palpation of the face, the tongue, the abdomen, the back, the voice, and the general demeanor of the patient. All these aspects can give clues to the appropriate treatment. A useful description of tongue diagnosis is given in the book *Modern Chinese Acupuncture* by G. T. Lewith and N. R. Lewith (published by Thorsons, 1980).

f. Specific note is made of any medication the patient is or has been taking as acupuncture has a chemical effect and this may be influenced adversely by medication (Rees, 1981).

Specific treatments

The following examples are a combination of recognized formulae for pain, my own experience in this field, and the experience of others. It could be regarded as a base for those with little experience in acupuncture or acupressure. If results are not satisfactory using these treatments, further reading is necessary.

A useful description of the location of the points is given in *An Outline of Chinese Acupuncture* referred to earlier (p. 134).

Stimulation with either acupuncture or acupressure is usually given on the side of the symptoms or bilaterally. In general, it is unwise to use more than five to ten points in any one treatment session.

Headache

Use the points in the area of symptoms. The appropriate points should be tender to deep palpation.

Frontal headache: gall bladder 14 and 20. colon 4
Temporal headache: three heater 3, 23. gall bladder 20
Occipital headache: gall bladder 20. governor vessel 15. bladder
                            10, 60.

Migraine

Treatment is of benefit both prior to, during, or between attacks. Again tender points are of greatest value: gall bladder 5, 6, 20. colon 4, 10

Chronic headache and migraine can be very successfully treated with acupuncture. Smirala (1981) reported on a study of treatment by acupuncture and/or manipulation on a group of 274 patients with chronic headache. His results showed that 84% of the group having only acupuncture had great improvement. 64% of the group having only manipulation showed the same degree of improvement. A further 45% of those in whom manipulation had no effect were improved considerably with acupuncture.

Liao (1980) reported on the acupuncture treatment of two hundred Caucasian patients with intractable head pain. Two thirds of these patients had pain duration of between 10 and 60 years with no demonstrable organic pathology. Complete relief of pain with no recurrence for at least two years and complete abstention of medication for a minimum of three months was achieved in 41.5% of patients. A further 35% had either substantial or complete pain relief and reduction of medication for between one week and three months.

Trigeminal neuralgia

Again choose tender points in the area of symptoms.

Opthalmic area: gall bladder 14. bladder 2. stomach 2. three
                          heater 5.
Maxillary area: stomach 2, 3, 44. governor vessel 26.

Mandibular area: stomach 6, 7, 44. conception vessel 24.

Kinoshita (1979) conducted a trial of treatment by acupuncture for this condition in 73 patients. He reports a cure in 71%, improvement in 25%.

Pain of cervical spine origin

Upper cervical spine: governor vessel 16, 20. small intestine 15. lung 7.
Lower cervical spine: governor vessel 16. three heater 10, 17, colon 4.
Whiplash: gall bladder 20. governor vessel 14
Torticollis: gall bladder 20, 39. small intestine 3.

Agrawal et al (1981) studied the effects of electroacupuncture on ninety cases of cervical spondylosis. Patients were treated for thirty minutes every day for ten days. Symptoms had been present in 85.5% of patients for over one year. Excellent results were achieved in 70% of the cases, good results in 20%.

Gunn and Milbrandt (1977d) report that acupuncture is extremely effective for the treatment of cervical spondylosis and that production of the Teh Ch'i phenomenon is important in achieving good results.

Shoulder pain

colon 16, 15, 14, 4. small intestine 10. three heater 14. (Fig. 5.4)
bladder 57. (Fig. 5.5)

I have found when improvement with acupuncture to the area of symptoms had ceased, that auricular acupuncture to the shoulder area of the ear produced a marked increase in range of movement and decrease of pain (Duffin, 1982).

Elbow pain

colon 11, 12, 4. three heater 10. gall bladder 34.

Gunn and Milbrandt (1977b) advocate needle insertion into tender points in the area of the elbow in types I to IV of tennis elbow (Cyriax classification). For type V, which they describe as having a cervical cause, they use additional points around the medial epicondyle, shoulder, arm, neck and hand. In the latter type, they

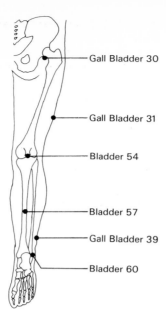

Fig. 5.5 Some commonly used points on the posterior aspect of the leg.

state that satisfactory relief of symptoms should occur within four to five weeks after the nerve roots are free, although if Wallerian degeneration has taken place recovery will take at least twelve weeks.

Acupuncture is not always successful in treating this kind of pain. I have had experience of one manual worker with a history of severe tennis elbow of duration in excess of six months. All forms of physiotherapy had been tried and failed. Acupuncture also showed no improvement.

Wrist pain

colon 4, 5. three heater 4, 5. lung 7, 9.

Dorsal spine pain

bladder 27, 45.

Herpes zoster

gall bladder 30, 31, 32, 42 and 43.

In a report of a study of eleven acute cases of herpes zoster Cordon (1976) describes excellent results in ten patients. Patients received both body acupuncture and auriculotherapy. One of the group was a child of three years of age, and in her case ultrasound was used as a means of stimulating the points. After one treatment, two patients had 100% pain relief, and two had 90% relief. After two treatments six had 100% pain relief and two had 75% relief. No further skin lesions occurred after commencement of treatment.

Superficial abdominal pain

conception vessel 7, 6. kidney 16, 17, 14.

I have used acupuncture to treat a patient with hypersensitivity and pain related to a laparotomy scar. The pressure of clothes on the scar was highly irritating. The patient had received only partial relief from an intercostal nerve block, and transcutaneous nerve stimulation had worsened her pain. On commencement of acupuncture treatment she estimated her pain as 65%. Initially, I used the above points, later including local sensitive spots within the scar. After two treatments, some pain reduction had been achieved and I used electrostimulation. After four treatments she estimated her pain as 20%. She was discharged after seven treatments describing her pain as 'negligible'.

Low back pain

bladder 23, 24, 25, 26, 27, 60.

It is possible that acupuncture for this condition, with or without sciatia, may be one of the most useful applications for physiotherapists.

Gunn et al (1980) report in a study of treatment by acupuncture for chronic low back pain (average 28 weeks duration) a clearly significant decrease in symptoms when compared with standard physical treatment. The 56 patients in his trial all received 8 weeks of physiotherapy, remedial exercises and occupational therapy without improvement. All patients continued with this regime but 29 randomly selected members of the group received acupuncture at motor points. All patients were reviewed at discharge, 12 weeks after discharge, and at approxiately 27 weeks. At all stages the group treated with acupuncture were significantly better than the controls. At final follow up 18 of the 29 acupuncture group had returned to their original employment, whereas in the control group of 27, only 4 had done so.

Mendleson et al (1983) conducted a placebo-controlled double-blind crossover trial of 77 self-selected patients suffering from chronic back pain. All patients had higher than normal depression, neuroticism and hypochondriases scores. The placebo treatment consisted of intradermal injection of 2% lidocaine into non-tender, non-acupuncture points in the lumbar area. Overall reduction in pain score was 26% for the acupuncture treated group, 22% for the placebo treated group: hence, the difference was not significant. On the other hand, Radwan (1981) quotes his results with acupuncture for low back pain as excellent or good in 90% of cases.

Sciatica

bladder 25, 31, 32, 33, 34, 51, 54, 60. Gall bladder 30, 34, 39 (Fig. 5.5).

When the pain distribution is posterior, bladder meridian points are found to be of most use. If the pain is lateral the gall bladder meridian points are the most appropriate. Radwan (1981) reports 37 excellent results out of a case-load of 50.

Hip pain

gall bladder 29, 30, 34.

I have had excellent results with two young (aged 18 and 21) female patients, A & B, with hip pain of undiagnosed origin. In both cases symptoms had been present over several months and all methods of physiotherapy treatment had failed.

Patient A had been admitted to hospital for investigation of an infective cause, but no such cause was found. Both patients complained of pain on all hip movements and on weight-bearing. In the case of patient A, the limitation of movement by pain was more severe.

I used the above gall bladder points with both cases, adding moxibustion and later electroacupuncture in patient B, who was less acute. In patient B needle penetration in gall bladder 30 was to a depth of approximately three inches.

Both patients responded well with decrease in pain and increase in range after each treatment. Patient A was discharged after four treatments and B after seven treatments.

Gunn and Milbrandt (1977a) report that on the investigation into 15 referred cases of diagnosed hip 'bursitis' they found that lumbar spondylosis was the cause of pain. While treatment should be directed to the spinal cause in these cases, relief of symptoms can be achieved by needle acupuncture into tender motor points around the hip.

Knee

Antero-medial pain. spleen 10, 9. liver 8, kidney 10.
Antero-lateral pain. stomach 34, 35, 36. gall bladder 34, 33.
Retro-patellar pain. extra point under the patella.
Posterior pain. bladder 54 (Fig. 5.5).

In my experience patients with knee pain show good results with acupuncture.

A manual worker aged 28, with X-ray changes showing early osteoarthritis, presented with constant knee pain aggravated by extremes of range. The area of pain fluctuated in its predominance and on each attendance I gave electroacupuncture to points close to the area of greatest pain. After each treatment complete pain relief occurred, demonstrable on examination by painfree over pressure. Pain relief lasted from 3 to 7 days following each treatment, and after 8 treatments the patient was symptom-free.

Another patient, whose anterior knee pain was limiting his attempts at knee mobilization, was given acupuncture to points in the painful area. This reduced his pain considerably within a few minutes, and made his mobilization much easier.

Ankle

Antero-lateral pain. stomach 41. gall bladder 40. bladder 60, 61, 62, 67.
Antero-medial pain. stomach 41. liver 3, 4. spleen 5. kidney 4, 5, 6.

As mentioned earlier I have found acupuncture to points around the lateral aspect of the ankle prior to friction massage to the lateral ligament very useful in increasing pain tolerance.

General applications

Various points are recognized for their value in relieving pain of a more generalized nature, e.g. three heater 5 coupled with gall bladder 41, when used bilaterally will help to relieve joint problems. Bladder 60 and liver 8 and colon 4 are useful for pain control in any area.

CAUTIONS AND CONTRAINDICATIONS TO ACUPUNCTURE

Sterilization

One of the possible complications of acupuncture is cross infection. Particular care is required with respect to hepatitis B. To avoid transference or introduction of infection, needles should be autoclaved prior to each use and the skin of the operator and patient should be cleansed with an antiseptic solution prior to handling or inserting the needle.

Forbidden points

There is a list of points which are traditionally forbidden to needle and/or apply moxa. All of these points lie close to important anatomical structures which should not be punctured. With expertise and experience most points can be needled but great care is necessary.

Debility and anxiety states

In general, debilitated or very anxious patients should not be given acupuncture, unless the latter wish to have such treatment for anxiety. Patients should never be persuaded to have acupuncture against their will. Acupressure in these cases may be a useful alternative.

Children

In general, acupuncture is not a suitable treatment for babies or children although there are exceptions. Acupressure in these cases may be of value.

Tumours

The area of, or close to, tumours of any type must not be needled.

Swellings

Swollen areas should not be needled unless the cause is known and is non-infective, e.g. sprained ankle.

Varicosities

These areas should not be given acupuncture.

Any severe skin lesions or areas of infection

Such areas should be avoided.

Menstruation

Patients may be treated during menstruation, although Nogier notes that some upset of the cycle may occur with auriculotherapy, and that the results of treatment tend to be less beneficial during this time.

Pregnancy

In general it is preferable not to treat a pregnant patient, especially if there is a history of threatened abortion. However, acupuncture is not contraindicated with the exception of points around the abdomen or breasts.

Acupuncture can be used to induce labour, to reduce labour pain and as a treatment for morning sickness and other minor complaints of pregnancy.

Sensitivity to acupuncture

The therapist should be aware that different patients have different reactions to acupuncture, varying from no response to immediate response with or without moderate degrees of euphoria or fainting.

One patient whom I treated for low back pain became euphoric for approximately 19 hours on each occasion following 20 minutes of treatment. During these 19 hours she described her emotional state as 'a high' and she did not feel safe to drive a car during this time. Her back pain resolved completely after 4 treatments.

Takeshige (1980) noted that the results of animal experiments showed that 25 times greater quantity of endogenous morphine-like factors were present in the brains of an acupuncture effective group of rats when compared to a group where acupuncture had no effect.

Pain as a warning

As with all pain-relieving modalities, it must be remembered that pain may be a necessary warning signal, and this factor must be carefully considered prior to commencement of treatment to alleviate pain.

RESEARCH

There is no doubt that acupuncture is useful in the relief of pain, although some patients are more susceptible to its effects than others. However, the existence of meridians and points is more difficult to establish, as is the mechanism by which acupuncture produces its effect.

Acupuncture research is in progress in almost all countries of the world and gradually scientific data, which to some extent explain its action, are accumulating.

Meridians

There is certainly some doubt about the existence of these channels as separate entities from nerve pathways. However, the Chinese mapped them on body charts long before Western medicine had established the course of nerves. It is possible that the meridian lines arose as a result of joining up points which were found to have a similar action.

Studies have been done in China, many of which demonstrate a sensation of numbness or 'running water' along the path of meridians following electroacupuncture (Academy of Traditional Chinese Medicine, 1979). This is referred to as propagated sensation along the channels (PSC). Its presence occurs more often in patients with pathology than in those without pathology.

A theory held by some researchers is that the meridians relate to the lymphatic system and blood vessels (Gong Qihua & Cao Jiren, 1981). However, Mann expresses the opinion that the speed with which a result can be achieved with acupuncture when applied to an area distal or contralateral to the area of pathology (1–2 seconds) excludes these systems as the pathways of conduction (Mann,

1977a). He feels the nervous system is the only means of conduction.

The 'inner pathway' connection between meridians and viscera corresponds to the dermatomal connection, and can be demonstrated by the cutaneo-visceral reflex. Kuntz et al in a series of experiments in 1940 showed that by stimulating the skin on the backs of animals, vascular changes occurred in the digestive organs corresponding to the dermatome stimulated (Mann, 1977a). Travell and Rinzler (1946) showed that by cooling trigger areas on the front of the chest with ethyl chloride, complete and prolonged relief of pain in angina pectoris or acute myocardial infarction ensued.

In 1979 at the National Symposium of Acupuncture, Moxibustion and Acupuncture Anaesthesia in Beijing, it was postulated that the meridian line and the nervous system may be identical (Guo Bangfu et al, 1979). However, Mann (1977c) describes how sometimes a needle inserted in the leg produces a sensation along the stomach meridian where it goes over the abdomen and thorax. This does not match a nerve trunk route.

An article published in the Chinese Medical Journal in 1983 describes four cases of spontaneous channel sensation all of which had intracranial pathology (Xue, 1983). The patients complained of linear sensations identical to the pathways of meridians. The author postulates the idea that there may be a meridian centre in the cortex.

Points

Many researchers equate acupuncture points with motor points (Gunn, 1978a). It is true that many correspond, but the number of described acupuncture points is in excess of the number of motor points.

Gunn classifies acupuncture points into four groups as follows:

Type I at motor points
Type II at focal meetings of superficial nerves in the sagittal plane
Type III at areas lying over superficial nerves or plexuses
Type IV at musculo-tendinous junctions (Gunn et al, 1976; Gunn, 1977)

His grouping was based on studies of 70 commonly used and effective points described by Matsumoto (1974), Mori (1977) and Mann (1966).

Many researchers have shown that acupuncture points are identifiable by measuring skin resistance to passage of an electric current (Nakatani, 1972, Saita, 1973). The areas are seen to be areas of low electrical resistance, although other researchers dispute this (Poon et al, 1980).

Plummer (1980) suggests that the relevance of perforating veins in the region of acupuncture points requires further documentation and study. It is his opinion that the individual irregularity of the sites of these veins may be the reason for failure of acupuncture therapy in some patients.

Lu et al (1981) have studied the composition of the nervous tissue underlying the acupuncture point stomach 36 in rats and compared it with a point 0.5 cm lateral to it. They found that there were more myelinated fibres, more large size fibres and more group II fibres at stomach 36 than at the nearby non-acupuncture point and suggest that these features may describe the basic characteristics of points.

Studies at the Physiology Institute in Shanghai have demonstrated more pressure receptors in the areas of acupoints, and at Sian Medical College the presence of more stretch receptors has been shown (Lu, 1983).

Teh Ch'i and needle grasp

Teh Ch'i phenomenon is a sensation felt by the patient within seconds following needle insertion into an acupuncture point. The sensation may be described as 'heaviness', 'numbness', 'tingling', 'fullness' or 'soreness'. Greatest pain relief is dependent on a patient experiencing this sensation.

The objective component of Teh Ch'i consists of the needle grasp phenomenon. Muscle spasm, local to the point of puncture, occurs and the needle appears to be drawn inwards into the tissues.

The sensation of Teh Ch'i is probably due to the stimulation of nociceptors, proprioceptors and interoceptors (Gunn & Milbrandt, 1977c).

Needle grasp may be superficial or deep (Gunn & Milbrandt, 1977c). The former will occur anywhere on the body with needle penetration of 1–2 mm and rotation of the needle. Deep needle grasp only occurs at type I acupuncture points, i.e. motor points.

Gunn explains that needle grasp is more obvious in patients who have hypersensitive receptors as a result of denervation supersensitivity. In these cases needle insertion and agitation causes great increase in the afferent barrage of impulses which produces intense local muscle contraction and needle grasp. In extreme cases the needle may be bent in situ (Gunn et al, 1976).

Effects

Acupuncture

Acupuncture has been shown by many researchers to have an analgesic effect (Lu Guowei et al, 1981). When the cardiac and cephalic ends of the carotid arteries of two animals are cross-connected, and one animal is given acupuncture, the pain threshold in both animals is found to increase.

Various theories of how acupuncture achieves analgesia have been suggested. At one time it was thought that it was merely stimulation of large diameter mechanoreceptors. Later, with the discovery of opiates and their increase following acupuncture, the theories altered to incorporate the new information. In 1975, Hughes and Kosterlitz discovered two chemicals which interacted with the same receptors as morphine and could produce significant analgesia. These chemicals were termed enkephalins, the most important of which appears to be methionine enkephalin. Several months later a larger endogenous opiate peptide, β-endorphin was discovered.

Since 1965 the Beijing Medical College Acupuncture Anaesthesia Research Group have accumulated evidence that acetylcholine, serotonin and endogenous opiate-like substances are all increased by acupuncture. In 1982 this research group published an article citing 5-hydroxytryptamine (serotonin) in the CNS as possibly one of the most important neurochemical agents in acupuncture analgesia (Han C-S et al, 1982).

Naloxone, an opiate receptor antagonist reduces or abolishes analgesia produced by manual or low frequency electroacupuncture (2–6 cycles per second) (Price & Rees, 1982). However it has no effect, in mice, on the analgesia produced by high frequency electroacupuncture (200 cycles per second). This suggests two different methods of pain relief and agrees with the observations of Zhang et al, (1980) which are that low frequency acupuncture may release β-endorphins and high frequency releases met-enkephalin.

A further theory of the mechanism by which acupuncture creates its effect relates to electrical field. In normal health a neuraxis has a positive electrical potential and the peripheral end of the nerve has a negative potential (Dowson, 1981). Under deep chemical anaesthesia these potentials are totally reversed. It is possible that electroacupuncture may also effect a reversal and in this way trigger off a chain of events which effects pathology.

Acupuncture anesthesia would appear to be mainly the result of sensory interaction within the CNS. Needle puncture results in afferent stimuli travelling via large and medium nerve fibres towards the cerebral cortex. This triggers off an inhibition of pain. It has been found that stimulation must be sufficiently above the threshold of medium sized fibres but that too strong a stimulus will activate the C fibres and will increase pain. The gate control theory of Melzack and Wall partly explains the mechanism of pain relief. The part played by the substantia gelatinosa and the thalamus provides further explanation. It appears that chemical neurotransmitters are fundamental in the analgesic effects of acupuncture.

Acupressure

It is probable that acupressure achieves its effect in a similar way to acupuncture.

In China, a comparison between patients undergoing subtotal gastrectomy while receiving either epidural anaesthesia or 'finger press anesthesia' has been reported (First Medical College of PLA, 1979). It was noted that those receiving epidural anaesthesia had a blood pressure (BP) drop of, on average, 18 mmHg which required post-operative medication in half the cases, whereas the 'finger press' group had an increase in BP of 20 mmHg which returned to normal spontaneously after operation. The gastrointestinal functions returned to normal after 29 hours post-operation in the finger press group, whereas this took 44 hours in the epidural group.

The same article also notes that both 'finger press' and electro-acupuncture can inhibit visceral stretching pain.

Dowson (1981) reports that a particular patient with migraine can abate an attack by deep acupressure on the area between the 1st and 2nd metatarsals, where liver 2 and 3 are situated.

Comparative studies

One of the major problems of scientific studies related to pain relief is the difficulty in measuring pain. Lewith and Machin have published a useful series of questionnaires related to the assessment of clinical effects of acupuncture, including pain relief (Lewith & Machin, 1981).

While there is a great deal of literature on the effects of acupuncture, there is considerably less on studies comparing its effects with those of other forms of physiotherapy.

Gunn et al (1980) have published a study comparing the results of acupuncture with 'standard physiotherapy' and report significantly better results with acupuncture.

Gunn (1978b) has also compared acupuncture and TNS for pain relief and found acupuncture of greater benefit. He explains this by the fact that the 'current of injury' in the case of acupuncture is constant and lasts for several days, i.e. while the microtrauma of puncture heals (Gunn, 1976). With TNS the current is exogenous and does not outlast the application of treatment.

Mendleson et al (1983) have compared the effects of acupuncture and placebo treatments in chronic back pain, and have found the difference to be not scientifically significant. However, their placebo treatment consisted of injection intradermally of 2% lidocaine into non-acupuncture points in the lumbar area and then inserting acupuncture needles superficially for 30 minutes. Gunn (1978a) maintains that this would result in an apparent barrage of nerve impulses which would be smaller than with a standard acupuncture procedure but could still result in some pain relief.

Smirla compared acupuncture with cervical manipulation for the treatment of headaches. He found more improvement with acupuncture.

A study by Berry et al (1980) comparing acupuncture, physiotherapy, steroid injection and oral anti-inflammatory therapy in shoulder cuff lesions showed marked improvement in almost all of sixty patients, with no significant difference between the effect of each type of treatment. The average duration of symptoms prior to the commencement of the study was 23 weeks. The authors' opinion was that perhaps none of the treatments had any effect and that, in view of the duration of symptoms prior to treatment, the good results may only have been due to natural recovery. They stress the significance of this possibility, as so many patients starting therapy have had similar duration of symptoms prior to treatment.

Fox and Melzack (1976) compared the effects of TNS and acupuncture in low back pain. They found that both methods produced a substantial decrease in pain, but neither was statistically better than the other. In my own experience I have found acupuncture to be of greater benefit, especially in cases where TNS has been of little use.

Dowson (1981) reported on the initial observations of sixty patients with osteoarthritis of the knee receiving treatment of physiotherapy or acupuncture. In both groups, 60% pain relief was achieved, but this occurred within three to four weeks of starting acupuncture, whereas in the group receiving physiotherapy it took ten weeks before pain reduction was noted. Dowson also notes that acupuncture is potentially less time consuming and cheaper than physiotherapy.

CONCLUSION

From this chapter I hope it is apparent that acupuncture is a huge topic. The more one reads about it the more one realises that there is much yet to learn. To quote Nogier, 'In life itself, and all the more so in medical life, we are absolutely sure of very little.' Perhaps that is the fascination of acupuncture.

More research is required, particularly in the comparative field. However, from the physiotherapy standpoint, I think the effort needs first to be placed on gaining expertise in acupuncture before considering acupuncture research. Very little work has been published on the effects of acupressure. Skill in acupressure could be achieved in a short period of time and studies could then be done comparing TNS or other pain relieving modalities with acupressure.

REFERENCES

The Academy of Traditional Chinese Medicine 1975 An outline of Chinese Acupuncture. Foreign Languages Press, Peking

Academy of Traditional Chinese Medicine 1979. Observation on phenomenon of propagated sensation along the channels. Advances in acupuncture and acupuncture anaesthesia. The Peoples Medical Publishing House, pp 21–22

Agrawal, Al, Rao Ravishankar R 1981 Cervical spondylosis: Treatment with acupuncture. British Journal of Acupuncture 4(1): 3–5

Berry H, Fernandes L, Bloom B, Clark R J, Hamilton E D B 1980 Clinical study comparing acupuncture, physiotherapy, injection, and oral anti-inflammatory therapy in shoulder-cuff lesions. Current Medical Research and Opinion 7(2): 121–126

Cho M H, Cho C 1978 A simple physiological method of isolating the topographical correspondence between somatic areas and auricular points, and the clinical application of this method for the pain treatment. Acupuncture & Electro Therapeutics Research International Journal 3: 113–120

Cordon N R 1976 Treatment of herpes zoster utilizing various acupuncture modalities. American Journal of Acupuncture 4(3): 257–262

Dowson D I 1981 Acupuncture in obstetrics. Newsletter of Association of Chartered Physiotherapists in Obstetrics and Gynaecology. Winter, pp 5–15

Duffin D H 1982 Acupuncture: results of nine months use in the National Heath Service. Physiotherapy 68(9): 298–300

First Medical College of PLA 1979 The study on finger press anaesthesia. Advances in Acupuncture and Acupuncture Anaesthesia, pp 205–206

Fox E J, Melzack R 1976 Transcutaneous electrical stimulation and acupuncture comparison of treatment for low-back pain. Pain 2: 141–148

Gong Qihua, Cao Jiren 1981 The relations between channels and lymphatic system. British Journal of Acupuncture 4(1):10

Gunn C C 1976 Transcutaneous neural stimulation needle acupuncture & 'Teh Ch'i' phenomenon. American Journal of Acupuncture 4: 317–322

Gunn C C 1977 Type IV acupuncture points. American Journal of Acupuncture 5(1): 51–52

Gunn C C 1978a Motor points and motor lines. American Journal of Acupuncture 6(1): 55–58

Gunn C C 1978b Transcutaneous neural stimulation, acupuncture and the current of injury. American Journal of Acupuncture 6(3): 191–196

Gunn C C, Milbrandt W E 1977a Bursitis around the hip. American Journal of Acupuncture 5(1): 53–60

Gunn C C, Milbrandt W E 1977b Tennis elbow and acupuncture. American Journal of Acupuncture 5(1): 61–66

Gunn C C, Milbrandt W E 1977c The neurological mechanism of needle-grasp in acupuncture. American Journal of Acupuncture 5(2): 115–120

Gunn C C, Milbrandt W E 1977d Shoulder pain, cervical spondylosis and acupuncture. American Journal of Acupuncture 5(2): 121–128

Gunn C C, Ditchburn F G, King M H, Renwick G J 1976 Acupuncture loci: a proposal for their classification according to their relationship to known neural structures. American Journal of Chinese Medicine 4(2): 183–195

Gunn C C, Milbrandt W E, Little A S, Mason K E 1980 Dry needling of muscle motor points for chronic low-back pain. Spine 5(3): 279–291

Guo Bangfu, Yao Zhiying, Zhang Qingcai, Shen Lei, Wang Liuqiang 1979 The clinical research on analgesic effect of acupuncture anaesthesia in lateral meniscectomy. Advances in Acupuncture and Acupuncture Anaesthesia, 202–203

Han C-S, Chou P-H, Lu C-C, Lu L-H ,Yang T-H, Jen M-F 1982 The role of central 5-hydroxytryptamine in acupuncture analgesia. British Journal of Acupuncture 5(2): 36–44

Hughes J, Smith T W, Kosterlitz H W et al 1975 Identification of two related pentapeptides from the brain with potent opiate agonist activity. Nature 258:577–9

Kinoshita H 1979 Mechanism and application of paraneural acupuncture for neuralgia. British Journal of Acupuncture 2(1):37

Lewith G T, Machin D 1981 A method of assessing the clinical effects of acupuncture. Acupuncture & Electro-Therapeutic Research International Journal 6: 265–276

Liao S J 1980 Use of acupuncture for relief of head pain. British Journal of Acupuncture 3(2):40

Lu G W 1983 Neurobiologic research on acupuncture in China as exemplified by acupuncture analgesia. Anesthesia and Analgesia 62:335–340

Lu Guowei, Xie Jingqiang, Yang Jin, Wang Yongning, Wang Qilin 1981 Afferent nerve fiber composition at point zusanli in relation to acupunture analgesia. Chinese Medical Journal 94(4): 255–263

Mabel M, Yang P, Kok S H, 1979 Further study of the neurohumoral factor endorphin in the mechanism of acupuncture analgesia. American Journal of Chinese Medicine 7: 143–148

Mann F 1966 Atlas of acupuncture. Heinemann, London

Mann F 1977a Scientific aspects of acupuncture. Heinemann, London, p 2

Mann F 1977b Scientific aspects of acupuncture. Heinemann, London p 32
Mann F 1977c Scientific aspects of acupuncture. Heinemann, London p 37
Matsumoto T 1974 Acupuncture for physicians. Charles C Thomas, Springfield,
    Illinois
Mendelson G, Selwood T S, Kranz H, Tim S L, Kidson M A, Scott D S 1983
    Acupuncture treatment of chronic back pain. A double-blind placebo-controlled
    trial. The American Journal of Medicine 74: 49–55
Mori H 1977 Modern acupuncture and moxibustion series. Soshichiro, Yokosuka,
    Japan
Nakatani Y 1972 A guide for application of ryodoraku autonomous nerve
    regulatory therapy. Japan (Private publication)
Nogier P M N 1972 Treatise of auriculotheraphy. Maisonneuve, Moulins-Lès-Metz,
    France
Omura Y 1978 Pain threshold measurement before and after acupuncture:
    Controversial results of radiant heat method and electrical method & the roles
    of ACTH-like substances & endorphins. Acupuncture & Electro Therapeutic
    Research International Journal 3: 1–21
Plummer J P 1980 Anatomical findings at acupuncture points. 3(2):39
Poon C S, Choy T T C, Koide F T, 1980 A reliable method for locating
    electropermeable points on the skin surface. American Journal of Chinese
    Medicine VIII(3): 283–289
Price P, Rees L H 1982 The chemical basis of acupuncture analgesia. British
    Journal of Acupuncture 5(2): 13–15
Radwan A M 1981 Acupuncture in Egypt. British Journal of Acupuncture
    4(2): 37–40
Rees L H 1981 Brain opiates and corticotrophin-related peptides. Journal of the
    Royal College of Physicians of London 2: 130–134
Saita H S 1973 Modern scientific medical acupuncture. Journal of American
    Osteopathic Association 72:685
Smirala J 1981 Acupuncture and vertebromanipulation in the treatment of
    headaches. British Journal of Acupuncture 4(2): 10–13
Takeshige C 1980 Individual effectiveness of acupuncture analgesia and
    endogenous morphine-like factors. British Journal of Acupuncture 3(2):38
Travell J, Rinzler S H 1946 Relief of cardiac pain by local block of somatic
    trigger areas. Proceedings of the Society for Experimental Biology and Medicine
    63: 480–482
Xue C-C 1983 Occurrence of spontaneous channel sensation in epileptic patients
    with intracranial damage. Chinese Medical Journal 96(1): 33–36
Zhang A, Pan X, Xu S, Sheng J, Mo W 1980 Endorphins and acupuncture
    analgesia. Chinese Medical Journal 93(10):673–680

Manual therapy: treat function not pain

EDITOR'S NOTE

In this chapter the author has presented his personal philosophy regarding the treatment of pain. It was originally intended that a second chapter presenting an opposing viewpoint should be included. Unfortunately this was not possible. However it is hoped that his chapter will provoke debate and discussion and stimulate further research.

INTRODUCTION

There are two very fundamental questions we need to ask ourselves before treating patients whose principal complaint is one of pain. First, do they in fact hurt as they say they do, and second, do we treat their complaint of pain or the underlying cause of pain?

In answer to the first question of do they in fact hurt, we have no choice but to accept the patient's statement as fact. Since it cannot be proved that a patient does not have pain when he says he does, there is no point in trying to determine his honesty. What we can do is to accept his statement and then set about trying to detect the physical reasons for his description of pain.

The second question concerning whether to treat the complaint of pain or the underlying cause can only be answered by stating that while we may seek to manage the pain we must address our attention to the cause of the pain. True, pain is what brings patients to us and it is from the pain that they seek relief. But it is the cause of pain that must be addressed, just as in a similar manner the treatment of an abdominal pain by the internist is directed not at relieving the pain but at correcting its cause.

These two premises, namely that we accept the patient's description of pain and treat the underlying dysfunction and not the pain, may seem so obvious that they barely warrant a chapter on this topic. This would be true were it not for the fact that a large number of clinicians do not practice in agreement with these premises.

All too often we question the patient's honesty (to no avail) and we treat pain until it is relieved and then proceed to discharge the patient without ever conducting an objective assessment of the underlying dysfunction or directing treatment at that dysfunction.

This is not likely to be the case in the treatment of the shoulder, in which both the patient and the therapist, in addition to being aware of the pain, are also aware of the movement restriction. Once the patient gains relief of pain, if there is still some movement restriction and that restriction is gradually decreasing, both the patient and the therapist will see the need to continue treatment as long as there is progress. But what of the lumbar spine? A painful low back is often treated by heat, massage and exercises until the relief of pain is achieved and then the patient is discharged! Instabilities or stiffness of the spinal segment, although detectable by a skilled clinician (Gonnella, 1982), usually remain undetected by inexperienced clinicians. Not knowing what is wrong, the clinician is content to discharge the patient once the complaint of pain has ceased. Out of the door goes the patient with one or more stiff or unstable segments still in need of treatment. It is no small wonder that the symptoms are very apt to recur at some later date when the degenerative process has advanced. Also, it is no small wonder that each time the patient returns for treatment the condition and the complaint both continue to worsen.

In my view it is time we treated the spinal joints like any other joint of the body by treating the cause of pain and continuing the treatment until an appropriate level of function has been restored. However not all therapists will share my view. For example Maitland (1960, 1968), a highly respected Australian therapist, places much of his emphasis on the treatment of pain and not on the treatment of function. He demonstrated his approach at a recent conference (Conference of the International Federation of Orthopaedic Manipulative Therapy, 1981), when he treated a patient who demonstrated bilateral but unequal limitation of shoulder abduction. Interestingly enough, the least limited shoulder was the most painful one. All week, he worked on the shoulder that was the least limited with stretching and oscillation procedures. As he proceeded with each treatment, he usually sought to see if what he was doing was decreasing the patient's pain—or the reproducibility of pain. At the end of the week, the progress of the patient was satisfactory both in terms of pain reduction and the increased range of motion. Then, from the audience a question was asked as to why he had not treated the other and more limited shoulder. Maitland replied that he had not treated it because the patient had not complained of it. I must admit to disagreement with this philosophy.

Obviously, we venture into murky waters if we claim that every stiff joint should be treated. However, we should also be aware that all patients with osteoarthritic hips that present with the complaint of pain would have shown, in the months and years preceding the onset of pain, an increasing degree of joint dysfunction. Could we, by the selection of appropriate manipulative and exercise procedures, have arrested and indeed reversed this trend to a painful osteoarthritis? I believe so.

EVALUATION OF PAIN

Where is your pain?
Please mark on the drawings below the areas where you feel your pain.

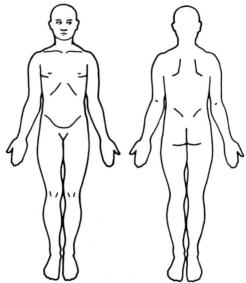

Fig. 6.1 Body chart (from Melzack, 1975)

Since I accept, without question, the patient's description of pain, it could be asked: what is there about pain that is left to evaluate? There is in fact a great deal to evaluate, particularly with regard to the patient's choice of words to describe the pain, both in terms of its character, its emotional effect and, of course, where it is felt.

People with pain find it difficult to be objective about it. After

There are many words that describe pain. Some of these are grouped below. Check (√) any words that describe the pain you have these days.

1.	2.	3.	4.
Flickering	Jumping	Pricking	Sharp
Quivering	Flashing	Boring	Cutting
Pulsing	Shooting	Drilling	Lacerating
Throbbing		Stabbing	
Beating	6.		8.
Pounding	Tugging	7.	Tingling
	Pulling	Hot	Itchy
5.	Wrenching	Burning	Smarting
Pinching		Scalding	Stinging
Pressing	10.	Searing	
Gnawing	Tender		12.
Cramping	Taut	11.	Sickening
Crushing	Rasping	Tiring	Suffocating
	Splitting	Exhausting	
9.			16.
Dull	14.	15.	Annoying
Sore	Punishing	Wretched	Troublesome
Hurting	Gruelling	Blinding:	Miserable
Aching	Cruel		Intense
Heavy	Vicious	19.	Unbearable
	Killing	Cool	
13.		Cold	20.
Fearful	18.	Freezing	Nagging
Frightful	Tight		Nauseating
Terrifying	Numb		Agonizing
	Drawing		Dreadful
17.	Squeezing		Torturing
Spreading	Tearing		
Radiating			
Penetrating			
Piercing			

Fig. 6.2 McGill pain questionnaire

all it is an unpleasant emotional experience. Pain has, however, innumerable characteristics: it may be local or referred, superficial or deep, hot or cold and so forth. Patients who are asked where their pain is, have little difficulty in describing where it began and to where it has spread, but they may forget that it is changing in distribution as well as in nature from day to day. The purpose of the body chart (Fig. 6.1) and the pain questionnaire (Fig. 6.2) is to capture at one particular point in time the patient's best description of their pain. Giving the patient these two forms to complete is, I have found, a far more accurate method of achieving a description of the patient's pain than by simply asking the question, 'How do you feel and where does it hurt?'. The use of words to describe recall of pain is limited at best. The patient's recall is frequently inhibited where he is faced by a professional person in a white coat. For this reason the patient is asked to complete the pain questionnaire and the body chart before his arrival in the clinic and before he even sees the clinician.

The pain questionnaire was developed by the McGill Group (Melzack, 1975) and has been found to be a worthwhile clinical tool. Two of the more significant lessons that I have learned from it are as follows:

1. Most patients who have minimal emotional stress from their pain do not mark words in such categories as 13 and 14, whereas those who have a severe or a relatively excessive emotional reaction to pain may mark words in categories 11 and 16.

2. Patients who mark a word or words anywhere in from 3 to 6 different categories usually progress at a satisfactory rate directly in proportion to the correction of their dysfunctions. However, those who mark 8 or more categories appear to have some emotional problems that hinder progress. Furthermore, if a patient marks 16 or more categories I have learned that I, acting alone, cannot help them. Clearly, they need psychological or psychiatric assistance as well as perhaps some physical therapy.

So valuable have I found the body chart and pain questionnaire that I use it on virtually every orthopaedic case that I see, except in the case of acute trauma where proceeding directly to treatment is more appropriate.

The emotional aspects of pain, particularly low back pain, cannot be ignored. Many of our patients start out with a low back pain, from a trivial or unknown cause, which gradually over a period of weeks increases in its magnitude. The patient's concern increases until a physician is consulted. Medication may not provide the relief desired and so a second and perhaps a third visit to the physician takes place. From here a referral may be made to the orthopaedic surgeon and either the physician or the surgeon may refer the patient directly to the physical therapist. At the point when the patient arrives to see the physical therapist, he does not have any great expectations of help from the therapist. Physicians are held highly in the esteem of patients. If they have been unable to help the patient then it may be unclear to him how someone who is not a doctor, and often younger, may be of assistance.

Whereas the pain started out on a purely physical basis, its emotional impact has since grown and the patient's ability to rationalize it as being of little consequence has been decreasing. Consequently, the three ring illustration in Figure 6.3(a), which

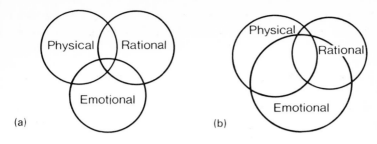

Fig. 6.3(a) This represents three aspects of pain. (b) This illustrates an overwhelming emotional concern, blocking out the physical and reducing the rational component.

describes the three aspects of pain, may have become somewhat distorted as illustrated in Figure 6.3(b).

The clinician clearly needs to be aware of the emotional component of the patient's disability. It is this emotional component that we should be treating from the very first contact with the patient. It is not difficult to treat if we begin by conducting a thorough evaluation of the rest of the patient's pain, not just by the picture of the body chart and pain questionnaire, but by the 10-step evaluation for dysfunction outlined in this chapter. When we are this thorough, we win the patient's respect concerning our interest, knowledge and skills. The patient, at the end of the evaluation, is ready to hear such statements as, 'There is nothing unusual here— we treat this type of condition all the time—you can expect relief after 8 to 12 treatments, depending on how well you tolerate the treatment and how well you do your home program.' At this most significant point in the therapist–patient relationship, the thoroughness of the evaluation and the consideration shown the patient by explaining the clinical findings paves the way in helping to erase the emotional overlay.

Of course, pain serves many useful purposes such as telling you to stop an activity, to change the posture or to move away from harm. Pain is, however, not a warning sign; it may be disproportionate to the pathology, may worsen when the condition improves, or may improve when the condition is worsening and continue when the pathology is long gone. These statements can be somewhat supported by the following observations:

1. Pain is not always a warning sign

You do not hurt until after you have been harmed, so pain does not truly serve as a warning sign. It is a symptom of something unpleasant, either physical or emotional, that has already taken place.

2. Pain is not in proportion to the severity of the pathology

Breast or other cancers may not hurt until they are well established to a degree that they may be terminal. If pain were a friend, if it were indeed a warning sign or if it were in proportion to the seriousness of pathology, then breast cancer should cause immediate and acute pain which unfortunately it does not. As a result, serious conditions may develop before they are noticed by the patient. On the other hand, the pain of a simple but unrelenting headache may be sufficient to drive some individuals to suicide. Pain is, therefore, not in proportion to the severity of the condition.

3. Lessening of pain does not always signal improvement

The first patient I ever treated complained of low back and leg pain and demonstrated a straight leg raising limitation. At each treatment session after traction he complained of less pain and the straight-leg raising showed improvement. At the end of two weeks, he was pain-free with a finding of 85 degrees for straight leg raising. I was extremely pleased until he related to me that over the past few days he had developed foot drop and was now beginning to stumble! Straight leg raising and his description of pain were purely subjective findings, having nothing to do with what was happening, i.e., a nerve root palsy.

4. Pain is affected by stimuli other than dysfunction

It is well known that the degree of pain which you experience is relative to the other stimuli that you are receiving. If, for instance, you are in pain at this moment, I can guarantee instant relief of your pain if I bring before you a submachine gun and discharge the magazine in your presence. The shock of my action would be sufficient to block any perception of pain that you have been experiencing. Likewise, a soldier charging up a hill in the heat of battle may be totally unaware that a bullet has entered his body, whereas at other times a simple pinprick would make him jump. Pain is relative to the other stimuli in our environment. Therefore, we acknowledge that factors such as inactivity, boredom, depression and perhaps even coffee may increase our pain whereas pleasurable activities, interests and a sensible diet may decrease it.

EVALUATION OF DYSFUNCTION

The cause of the pain will either be in the presence of a disease or of a dyfunction. Since it is the physician's role to exclude or identify disease, it remains for us to evaluate and later treat dysfunction. In order to do this we must have an appropriate grounding in such subjects as biomechanics, pathology and dysfunction. Cyriax (1982) in his textbooks on orthopaedic medicine (which I would retitle *Orthopaedic Dysfunction*) has provided an invaluable insight into the cause, evaluation and treatment of the muscle skeletal system. His work on evaluation of the extremities is a must for the physical therapist who treats extremity conditions. I would, however, disagree with Cyriax in most of his views concerning the spine, particularly his view that the intervertebral disc is the main culprit and that it can be easily influenced by manipulation and traction. In my view manipulation and traction, which I strongly endorse, are more likely to effect relief when symptoms come from the facet joints, myofascia and the sacroiliacs rather than from the intervertebral disc.

There are 11 steps which should be followed in evaluating extremity dysfunction and these may be listed as:
1. Pain assessment
2. Initial observation of functions—gait, sitting, etc.
3. History—interview
4. Structural and postural inspection
5. Active movements and end-feel of joints
6. Neurological assessment
7. Palpation for condition, position and mobility of joints
8. Consideration of radiographics and other reports
9. Summary of objective findings
10. Plan of treatment
11. Expected outcomes or prognosis

It is not my purpose to discuss each of these steps in detail here but an awareness of them is important.

There is, however, one aspect of the evaluation which is the most significant when it comes to evaluating extremity dysfunction and that is the topic of 'end-feel'. End-feel is the quality of resistance that can be elicited passively by the clinician when moving a joint to the end of its range. All joints have a characteristic end-feel, distinctive to the structure being stressed, and will differ at the end of ranges in the same joint—and even between individuals.

Cyriax (1982) describes three normal end-feels, whereas I choose to describe five (Paris, 1980):

1. Soft tissue approximation:
   soft and spongy
   e.g. elbow or knee flexion
2. Muscular:
   elastic reflex resistance with discomfort
   e.g. hamstring stretch
3. Ligamentous:
   firm arrest of movement with no give or creep
   e.g. abduction of the extended knee
4. Cartilagenous:
   sudden stop but not hard
   e.g. extension of the elbow
5. Capsular:
   firm arrest of movement with a slight creep
   e.g. steady hyperextension at the elbow

PHILOSOPHY OF TREATMENT

There is no one single approach to the treatment of dysfunction that is clearly superior to all others. Between the philosophies of those therapists who concentrate on pain relief and mine which emphasises the need for restoration of function, there are any number of personal approaches—most of which are no doubt valid. We must each acquire our own personal treatment philosophy based on our educational, experiential and private perception of patients' needs. Out of this we each develop a treatment philosophy or, if you wish, a personal bias. My personal philosophy may be summed up in the following eight statements:

1. Joint injuries, including such conditions referred to as osteo-arthritis, instability and the after-effects of sprains, are not diseases but dysfunctions.

2. Dysfunctions are manifested as either increases or decreases of motion from the expected normal or by the presence of aberrant movements. Thus, dysfunctions are represented by abnormal movement.

3. Where the dysfunction is detected as limited motion, the treatment of choice is mobilization (manipulation) of joint struc-

tures, stretching of muscles and fascia, and the promotion of activities that encourage a full range of movement.

4. When the dysfunction is manifested as increased movement, laxity, or instability, the treatment is not mobilization of the joint in question, but stabilization by instruction concerning correct posture, stabilization exercises, and correction of any limitations of movement in neighboring joints that may contribute to the need for compensation.

5. Degenerative joint structures, such as cartilage and ligaments, may be made to regenerate by such methods as altering alignment, reducing impact loading, providing frequent low-load use and by removing myofascial and capsular restrictions, improving postural alignment and instructing in correct use.

6. The physical therapist's primary role is in the evaluation and treatment of dysfunction, whereas that of the physician is the diagnosis and treatment of disease.

7. In this age where in some medical schools the study of the anatomy of the extremities is elective, and where spinal dissection is rarely required, physical therapists have the added responsibility of developing their knowledge of the structure and function of the neuro-muscular-skeletal system so that they may safely assume the leadership in the conservative treatment and management of this system.

8. The clinician, while being a good listener and demonstrating appropriate humility, must also offer reassurance and confidence about her own ability in order that the patient's emotional concerns are managed and the instructions followed. A clinician, although frequently in error, should not present herself as being in doubt.

PAIN MANAGEMENT

Although my emphasis is on the treatment of the dysfunction and not the pain, the patient, not infrequently, may need to have assistance in coping with the pain. At such times, heat, transcutaneous electrical nerve stimulation, acupressure and other modalities including oscillatory motion, either active (Codman, 1934), or passive (Maitland, 1968; Maitland, 1980), may help. For most other complaints of pain which are not acute, my approach is best described as belonging to the discipline of behavioral modification. I feel quite strongly that it is up to us whether we wish to reinforce and encourage the patient's perception of pain or whether we wish to focus the patient's attention away from his pain and towards more objective behaviors in terms of functional improvements.

I began by measuring the patient's desire to have due attention paid to his pain. This is achieved by having the patient complete the pain questionnaire and body chart. Next, by completing a thorough evaluation along the lines already outlined, we raise the patient's awareness of the underlying causes of his pain. This is particularly true if, during the evaluation, we 'find the spot' by palpation and 'reproduce the pain' by selective tension and other procedures.

There are, however, an additional number of concerns which relate to day-to-day management.

1. Turning the patient toward function

Before seeing the patient, a quick glance at the completed questionnaire will save many minutes of questioning regarding the pain.

After completing my examination, which includes the history, structure, active and passive movements, palpation for condition and position, etc., I outline to the patient my findings of dysfunction and ask the question, 'Tell me, please, what troubles you the most, your pain or your loss of function?' If this were the first question of the examination, the patient would inevitably respond that the pain was of paramount concern. Occasionally, by now, the examination has revealed to the patient several areas of altered function, knowledge of which may have already changed the patient's attitude from one of primary concern about pain to concern about function. If, however, as is usually the case, the patient responds that it is the pain that concerns him most, then I reply, 'That is quite understandable but do you now appreciate that your pain is a result of your problems and do you understand that I shall be treating your problems and not your pains?' They invariably do understand and we are off to a good start.

2. The second greeting

At the next visit, the philosophy that we are treating dysfunction and not pain must be reinforced from the very outset. No one on the staff, professional or clerical, is allowed to greet the patient by such statements as, 'Good morning, how are you?' Asking a patient how they feel as an opening question, no matter how well intended, will only focus the patient's attention on their pain and not on their objective functional improvement. Instead of the previous greeting, try one such as, 'Good morning, please come with me and I'll check on your progress.' Then, after a thorough reassessment of the patient's objective clinical findings and an explanation of their progress or regression, I ask the patient, 'And by the way, how have you been feeling?'

3. Make treatment visits condition-dependent, not pain-dependent

Some patients like coming for treatment; it is a social highlight, a validation that something is indeed wrong. If on reporting that they are feeling better, you respond, 'Then, I won't need to see you tomorrow', they may sense a disinterest, an isolation or even a punishment for having said that they are feeling better and, as a result, may immediately begin to demonstrate pain behaviour in order to get your sympathy and have you continue seeing them. They do this to manipulate you, in order that you do not reduce their visits. Incidentally, they are often effective in managing it!

From the beginning, the physical therapy treatments are not to be dependent on pain reduction. The dose is decided by the condition and not the complaint and this is exactly the way that medications should also be dispensed. Complaints of pain should not be rewarded by an increase in visits, and a decrease in pain response should not be punished by decreasing the visits. Patients do not like being handled that way. Instead, from the very outset the therapist should make it clear to the patient that he will be seen for a specified number of times over a specified number of weeks, for example, three times a week for three weeks. The schedule is then maintained unless there is a real and solid reason why the treatment should be either increased or decreased. Remember when undertaking treatment to restore function rather than pain you can, with practice, be reasonably sure as to how long the treatment programme will take. It is much more difficult to estimate this when working to relieve pain.

4. Do not enhance pain memory

Every time you perform an action that hurts, the structure becomes more sensitive and the pathway for conducting the pain is facilitated so that next time it will hurt more easily, even if a reduced stimulus is given. Not only have the structure and pathways changed, but the patient also begins to associate the action or movement with pain. Soon he will show all the emotional responses that the pain caused, although a cause for the pain may no longer exist. This situation is termed 'pain memory' and occurs as a direct response to the repeated association between cause and effect.

5. Turn off pain behavior

There are numerous little considerations that go into the behavioral approach, some of which have been outlined above. One addition is my approach to the patient who, on making eye contact, demonstates pain when, for instance, rising from a chair but does not demonstrate such pain when he is unaware that I am observing him. With this patient I would turn away from his pain behavior and not allow him to see that I have observed it. I then take the first opportunity to show approval and shower praise upon him when he does not demonstrate pain during a similar activity. I give him warmth and love for positive behavior and nothing for negative pain behavior. My patients are not my children but at times need to be treated as such.

6. When to treat pain rather than dysfunction

In acute conditions where pain predominates, the degree of protective muscle holding inhibits the return of normal function. In this situation we must treat the pain by whatever means at our disposal in order to remove the muscle holding and so allow for the return of function. Of course, in these cases the presence of pain takes precedence over the restoration of function. The supportive modalities for this I have already outlined. But be careful. Before removing protective muscle guarding make sure there is no underlying and continuing cause for which the muscle holding is serving a useful purpose, such as in the case of a recent fracture.

7. What if we increase pain during treatment?

There are times when we should be careful not to aggravate the pain, but there are also occasions when it really does not matter if we do. There are even times when it is absolutely necessary to increase pain.

In most acute states we should avoid aggravating the pain unless there is a positional fault that needs correction, such as a displaced meniscus at the knee, or a sacroiliac joint or facet that has locked out of position.

In the non-acute condition there are also occasions when it may be necessary to hurt our patients. Examples are many and include stretching out of shoulder capsules and the application of transverse frictions (Cyriax, 1982). On occasion, our treatments may aggravate the pain to such a degree that it may radiate into one of the limbs. An example may be in the correction of an acute lumbar kyphosis. Here, we first need to determine from the patient's history and lack of neurological signs whether or not the condition is arising from the intervertebral disc or from other structures such as the facet or muscles. If the disc is not involved it becomes important to force the patient out of their forward bent position and back into the neutral position. Such forcing may cause acute discomfort with radiation of pain, but if we are convinced that we are not aggravating any serious pathology but only forcing the spine into a more correct and better position which will enhance recovery, we should continue.

TREATMENT OF DYSFUNCTION

It will be seen from the section on philosophy that I consider dysfunctions to take many forms including a restriction of motion. Restrictions of motion represent perhaps the most common dysfunction and usually indicate the need to provide movement. For if a joint remains limited in range:
1. the capsule will continue to lose its extensibility (Akeson & Wayne, 1961).
2. without the stimulus of normal movement, the collagen remodelling will alter the normal capsular make-up, promoting yet further stiffness and loss of extensibility (Akeson et al, 1977).
3. the synovial lining will proliferate into the joint space, smothering that area of the cartilage no longer in use. Fibrous adhesions then begin to destroy the joint surface (Enneking & Horowitz, 1972).
4. the stiff joint which has lost its joint play motion is more prone to injury, because beyond its active range there is little if any tolerance to an outside force. Such a force will usually result in further injury (Mennell, 1964).

When we wish to promote motion, we need to consider the subject of end-feel. Nine abnormal end-feels which serve to limit the range of motion are listed below. These are labelled according to the structure which I feel is most likely to be at fault. Each is followed by a brief statement describing how I would treat it (Paris, 1980).

1. Capsular—proportionate in characteristic pattern (Cyriax, 1982).
   a. chronic inflammatory—harsh, tight arrest, characteristic of fibrosis. Treatment: heat and stretching
   b. acute inflammatory—painful with induced muscle guarding. Treatment: mild heat or ice and oscillations
2. Adhesions and scarring—sudden sharp arrest in one direction, common in the knee. Treatment: stretching or a high velocity thrust manipulation
3. Bony block—sudden hard stop short of normal range such as myositis ossificans or fracture within a joint. Treatment: none
4. Bony grate—rough, raw, cervical facets, advanced chondromalacia. Treatment: repreated low load, high frequency motion (continuous passive motion)
5. Springy rebound—cartilage block/meniscus, subluxated meniscus at the knee. Treatment: manipulation
6. Pannus—soft crunchy squelch, common in elbow on extension. Treatment: repeated active motions stopping just short of the squelch
7. Loose—ligamentous laxity, hypermobile type, rheumatoid. Treatment: If rheumatoid, then support and posture. If not rheumatoid, frequent low stimulus stretches to the ligaments
8. Empty—boggy, soft, not limited mechanically, characteristic of synovitis and haemarthrosis. Treatment: synovitis—rest, elevation and compression; haemarthrosis—aspiration
9. Painful—considerable pain before end of range is reached. End-feel is thus lacking in resistance other than the patient's protective or evoked splinting or spasm. Suspect disease including neoplasm, bursitis, abscess. Treatment: provide pain relief without joint stress, e.g. TENS, acupressure

A knowledge of end-feel is invaluable in the evaluation of extremity dysfunction. In the spine, end-feel is of limited value but nonetheless significant when present. Effective treatment of the spine is very dependent on a sound biomechanical knowledge as well as an awareness of the many syndromes that may be present.

SUMMARY

In this chapter I have not set out to prove my philosophy of treating dysfunction rather than pain, for philosophies resist such proof. Rather, I have tried to illustrate my philosophy and explain how I implement it. If you are currently treating pain rather than dysfunction and discharging patients when they are no longer complaining of pain rather than objectively assessing their physical findings, then I encourage you to consider that my approach might have something more to offer your patient than simply their relief of pain—it might prevent recurrences.

REFERENCES

Akeson W H, Wayne H 1961 An experimental study of joint stiffness. Journal of Bone and Joint Surgery 43-A: 1022–1034
Akeson W H, Amiel D, Mechanic G L et al 1977 Collagen cross linking alterations in joint contractures changes in reducible cross-links in periarticular connective tissue collagen after nine weeks of immobilization. Connective Tissue Research 5.1: 15–19
Codman E A 1934 The shoulder. Thomas Todd, Boston
Conference of the International Federation of Orthopaedic Manipulative Therapy 1981. Chridekech, New Zealand
Cyriax J H 1982a Textbook of orthopaedic medicine, vol I Bailliere Tindall, London
Cyriax J H 1982b Textbook of orthopaedic medicine, vol II Bailliere Tindall, London
Enneking W F, Horowitz M 1972 The intra-articular effects of immobilization on the human knee. Journal of Bone and Joint Surgery 54-A, 5: 973–985
Gonnella C, Paris S V, Kutner M 1982 Reliability in evaluating pressive intervertebral motion. Physical Therapy 62(4): 436–444
Maitland G D 1968 Vertebral manipulation. Butterworths, London
Maitland G D 1980 Peripheral manipulation. Butterworths, London
Melzack R 1975 The McGill pain questionnaire: major properties and scoring methods. Pain 1(3): 277–99
Mennell J 1964 Joint pain. Little Brown, Boston
Paris S V 1980 Course notes: extremity dysfunction and mobilization. Institute Press, Boston, Massachusetts
Paris S V 1983 Spinal manipulative therapy. Clinical Orthopaecics and Related Research (179): 55–61

Manual therapy: treat function and pain

I. MANUAL THERAPY AS PART OF AN INTEGRATED APPROACH TO PHYSICAL THERAPY TREATMENT OF PAIN

The practice of manual therapy has taken different courses in the various parts of the world and also among the individual physical therapists (Cookson, 1979; Cookson & Kent, 1979). Treatment methods mainly based on biomechanical principles, such as joint mobilization/manipulation, and methods mainly based on neurophysiological principles, such as PNF (Knott & Voss, 1968), Rood (Heiniger & Randolph, 1981; Stockmeyer, 1969), and Bobath (Semans, 1967), can be combined to the benefit of the individual patient. It is also my experience that Connective Tissue Massage (Teirich-Leube, 1978) is a valuable tool when testing and treating patients with joint dysfunction and pain.

This article is an attempt to show how all these methods can be integrated in order to reduce pain by improving or restoring function.

I will take examples from patients with dysfunction in the extremities. The clinical problems these patients represent are complex. Several structures in and around the joint may be at fault, and the dysfunction is often not localized to only a single joint or extremity or to one part of the spine. The rest of the body will also be affected, which means that the whole patient must be treated, and one must remember that the psyche cannot be dissociated from the soma.

Clinical experience has shown me that patients with pain and joint dysfunction cannot be treated by any one method alone. When function is impaired, there is usually both an arthrogenic and neuromuscular component, and almost always an accompanying pain component. The autonomic aspect needs to be emphasized when there is an increase in sympathetic tone.

Kaltenborn (1980) uses the term manual therapy about the evaluation and treatment of joints and their surrounding structures in order to relieve pain, increase or decrease mobility. It also includes teaching the patient possible ways to prevent the recurrence of the dysfunction.

Manual therapy, as expressed here, is much more than testing of joint play, and restoring it when it is limited or lacking. Joint manipulation is an important part of manual therapy, but it can never be practiced alone when the goal is to restore function.

Perhaps one of the reasons why manual therapy is practiced differently by different physical therapists is that they have a variety of points of view on the following questions:
— What does normal function demand of the body as a whole and of one specific joint?
— Is the joint looked upon as:
   a biomechanical structure?
   a receptor?
   or both?

A. Normal function

Normal function requires interaction of the whole body. It demands balance between mobility and stability. Normal function can also be defined as normal coordination. We do not think of coordination in relation to one muscle or one joint, but in relation to functional movement.

What does a coordinated movement look like?
— it has a purpose
   normal timing, speed and precision
   normal range of motion with normal joint play
— it is economical
— it can be alternated
— it has an adequate reflex base.

The motor system is often looked upon as two parts:
1. the peripheral part: the joints and the muscles
2. the central part: the control system—the nervous pathways.

We will be very limited in our therapeutic thinking and possibilities if we consider the joints and the central nervous system as separate entities. The unified concept is a *must*. First, each part will be regarded separately. Under the section on evaluation and treatment in this chapter, their interaction will be evident.

Since the understanding of normal function is closely linked to the appreciation of what takes place in the joint itself during movement, I will stress this in some detail. In all extremity joints there is normally present a characteristic amount of passive translatoric gliding and traction (joint play). These passive movements can be performed provided the joint is in a loose-packed position. When the bone is moved actively or passively, a roll-gliding takes place in the joint. Roll-gliding is a movement composed of rolling and gliding. Rolling is a movement where new points on one articular surface come in contact with new points on the other surface. Gliding is a movement where one point of the joint surface comes in contact with new points on the other surface. The combination of simultaneous rolling and gliding movements of articular surfaces increases the effective range of movement in the joint. With gliding or rolling alone, such a range could only be achieved by considerably more extensive articular surfaces.

The direction of the individual movements, rolling and gliding, varies according to the anatomical structure of the moving joint surface, i.e. whether it is concave or convex. If a bone motion takes place in one direction, the rolling that accompanies the movement takes place in the same direction.

The gliding in the joint, which accompanies the motion, takes place:

1. in the opposite direction if the moving joint partner is convex
2. in the same direction if the moving joint partner is concave
   (Kaltenborn, 1980).

In order for normal movement to take place, the rolling and gliding movements must occur at the right time and in the right amount. If not, joint play is limited, lacking or excessive; function will be impaired, and most likely associated with pain. A minor dysfunction, for example limited joint play in one of the small joints of the wrist, will cause pain and dysfunction of the patient's movement pattern. It is necessary to acquire a three-dimensional view of the joints, in order to understand this combination of gliding and rolling in the different joints (Williams & Warwick, 1980; Kaltenborn, 1980).

As therapists, we should be able to distinguish between the several factors that influence and may disturb the normal movement pattern.

The ligaments and the capsule limit and guide movement. Together with the muscles they maintain the integrity of the joint. In order to have normal control of movement and posture, information is needed from the periphery. Integration of stimuli from receptors in the joints, ligaments, fatpads and muscles, together with input from the eyes and equilibrium receptors, provide this information. Interaction is also needed from central control systems. We need the integration of righting, protective and equilibrium reactions in order to control movement and posture.

An example of how disturbed afferent information produces a general dysfunction in the motor system is described by Freeman et al (1965) in their classical article. They have shown how sprained ligaments of the ankle affect the function of the body as a whole. The instability of the foot the patient complains about is not only due to the weakening of the ligaments but also to the lack of sensory input from the structures in and around the joints. This influences the innervation pattern to the muscles in the vicinity of the joint and incoordination is the result. The patient's balance on the extremity is impaired; he gets a feeling of the foot giving way, and it does not react properly when walking on uneven ground. A local lesion has generated a general dysfunction in the motor system.

Motor reactions needed to get away from a stimulus must be quick enough in order to be adequate, and reactions that call for stability functions must be maintained in order to be normal. The anticipation of a movement and adjustment of posture to movement is called 'a postural set' by Bobath.

Muscle function is to develop and sustain tension. There is a balance of muscle strength between agonists and antagonists, and also within the various synergies. A coordinated movement has timing; there is a normal sequence of muscle contractions in any motor activity. Muscles that are mainly phasic and muscles that are mainly tonic interact so that the movement is controlled. The muscles should be able to:

— initiate a movement
— maintain a contraction against resistance
— work in a co-contraction pattern, both weight-bearing and non-weight-bearing with and without movement.

Muscle strength in a dynamic activity must not be equated with the muscular stability needed to do the controlled eccentric contractions while walking on uneven ground, or lowering the arm from overhead while holding something heavy.

Movements associated with pain, whether it is of mechanical or chemical origin, will be impaired. A patient will try to avoid putting weight on a painful extremity, and refrain from anything that hurts. Pain is a major inhibiting factor and a strong sympathetic stimulus, and cannot be ignored. This must also be kept in mind when evaluating and treating patients with joint dysfunction and pain.

B. Common denominators in an integrated approach

When considering such a variety of approaches for evaluation and treatment of patients, it is necessary to establish some common denominators. These are:
1. stimulus–response
2. need–supply
3. mobility–stability.

We can translate our various methods into *types of stimuli* which makes them easier to combine (Stockmeyer, 1969). This will broaden our understanding concerning the application of manual therapy procedures as well as the other techniques. Each technique will stop being good or bad when we consider the types of stimuli that one specific activity might generate. It will be much easier to adapt the technique to the individual patient, so that it is not absolutely necessary to perform specific movements or procedures in the *one* and *only* correct manner in order to be *right*. It is always the therapist's application and adaptation of the chosen method to the individual patient that counts.

We must look for the *patient's reaction to our handling*—observe the immediate reactions, but also be aware of the latency effects of our intervention. There will always be alternatives, both to the methods chosen and to the sequence in which we apply them. This makes integration of approaches challenging. Part of our evaluation will therefore be to identify the types of stimuli the patient needs. Our treatment ought to produce some of these stimuli in order to be effective. This implies that we need to speak a therapeutic language that the patient's body and mind appreciates and understands, and that we carefully observe the response to our intervention. It also implies that we select procedures that restore the homeostasis in the body, or at least not increase the imbalances.

We, as therapists, are not *ruled* by our methods and techniques. These are tools that we must handle *sufficiently well* in order to have enough specific tests and stimuli to apply when needed. Any person will respond to stimuli from his external or internal environment. The reactions may be autonomic, motor or psychosocial. Any stimulus may give any of these reactions. The whole treatment situation—including the therapist's own behaviour—is a stimulus that affects the patient. The patient must always be understood in view of his physical dysfunction and psychosocial background.

The locomotor system needs an integration of mobility and stability both in relation to joints and to muscle function. Mobility and stability are not in contrast to each other, they are mutually related. Some of the terms related to joints need to be defined:

— hypomobility: the joint has less range of motion (ROM) than normal

— hypermobility: the joint has greater ROM than normal around a physiological axis

— pathological hypermobility: when hypermobility is associated with pain

— instability: the joint has a lack of stability due to:

    a. ROM is greater than normal around an axis that is not physiological, either in a normal or abnormal movement plane.
Lack of muscular stability is often combined with instability in the joint itself.

    b. ROM is less than normal due to limited gliding and consequently the joint is unable to get into the closed-packed position.
If movement is forced beyond the range where the gliding is normal, the movement axis is shifted from its normal position, often in the direction of the periphery of the joint.
Compression develops at this point of the joint, together with stretch of the ligaments and the capsule on the opposite side.

The clinical signs that the patient presents to us can be seen as change in mobility/stability. A patient with a rupture of the cruciate ligaments in the knee will have lack of stability, whereas a patient who has suffered a fracture of the femur 3 months ago, and just had his plaster removed, will most likely have a decreased mobility in the affected extremity. He will also have lack of stability.

When practicing manual therapy it is of utmost importance to recognize when a joint with limited range of motion also has a *hidden instability* in the same joint. A patient with dysplasia of the hip has such a hidden instability in the joint. Another example is a patient who has limited range of motion in the shoulder secondary to an injury, such as a partial rupture of the rotator cuff.

These patients need to be treated differently than those who have limited joint play as the main cause of the restricted movement and pain. As mentioned, patients with degenerative joint diseases have an impairment of both mobility and stability, and usually there is an arthrogenic and neuromuscular component. The arthrogenic component is related to the degree of joint play. The neuromuscular component is related to the development of phasic and tonic functions (Heiniger & Randolph, 1981; Stockmeyer, 1967).

II. EVALUATION OF PATIENTS WITH PAINFUL JOINT DYSFUNCTION

In several textbooks, excellent schemes for patient evaluation are presented, and I refer to a few of these (Cookson & Kent, 1979; Maitland, 1977; Polly & Hunder, 1978).

I will mention some of the procedures to show how manual therapy can be combined with other approaches in the evaluation of patients with painful joint dysfunction (Ellingsen, 1981).

In everyday life in the clinic, evaluation must be performed without sophisticated technical equipment; we have to rely on what we see, hear and feel. The evaluation starts with estimating the activity in the patient's autonomic nervous system in order to decide how much stimulation the patient might tolerate, such as movements, handling and resistance—especially in relation to testing of passive translatoric movements. This is particularly important when the patient is experiencing pain and anxiety.

I listen carefully to how the patient describes his own problems:
— How does he assess his own condition?
— Does he have pain? Have him explain the location, duration and intensity of the pain. Is it related to movement or maintaining of positions?
— Is more than one joint affected?
— Does the extremity feel stiff or heavy?
— How is the sensation on the affected extremity for touch and temperature? Does the water in the bathtub, for example, feel differently on the two extremities?

I observe the patient's posture and movement patterns:
— How does he perform the activities of daily living?
— Does he have normal balance reactions?
— Are there any spontaneous movements of the affected extremity or does he protect it?

Since the patient's autonomic nervous system often is pushed toward the sympathetic side, clinical signs such as sweating, oedema, colour, skin and temperature changes are noted. The respiration pattern, pupils and general behaviour may also give an indication of the present state. A total evaluation of the Connective Tissue Zones on the patient's back is relevant in cases where a number of signs of increased sympathetic tone are present in addition to pain.

A patient with several indicators of increased sympathetic tone and severe pain should be recognized by the therapist as a candidate for reflex sympathetic dystrophy, and be treated as such, even though the medical diagnosis is not yet given. This patient should not be subjected to any further evaluation at this point. The first goal for our intervention is already evident: try to dampen the activity in his sympathetic nervous system and reduce pain. A possible outline of alternatives is given under treatment planning. To continue the evaluation, general mobility tests are done actively as a screening examination.

Finally, the affected joints are assessed for active and passive range of motion, including 'end-feel' and joint play. The relevant movements are tested for coordination, strength and stability. PNF, with its patterns of facilitation and different techniques, is a valuable tool when evaluating normal timing of movement and stabilizing functions. Muscle length is estimated by carrying the extremity passively through related PNF-patterns, if these movements are not, for some reason, contraindicated. Are the short muscles strong and hypertonic, leaving the antagonists weak and elongated? Palpation of the muscles and the skin will determine if they are adherent to the underlying structures. Cyriax (1975) has described how to differentiate pain arising from the joint itself, or the surrounding structures, and offers in his book wide knowledge in diagnosing soft tissue lesions.

In short, when active and passive movements are restricted and painful in the same direction, it is most likely an arthrogenic lesion. When the active and passive movements are restricted and painful in the opposite direction, it is most likely a soft tissue lesion.

When the limitation of motion is according to a capsular pattern, the movements of joint play are tested. Traction is always done first, then gliding and compression. These tests are described and portrayed in Kaltenborn's book (1980), *Mobilization of Extremity Joints*.

The route taken in the evaluation of a patient may take us along a variety of roads. This, of course, is not possible to predict. Our findings ought to agree with the patient's complaints and give us a tentative answer to the following questions:
— What is wrong?

— How did it get that way?
— What can be done about it?

III. TREATMENT OF PATIENTS WITH PAINFUL JOINT DYSFUNCTION

The planning process is based on the patient's history and all the information the evaluation has given.

I will discuss three patient examples in order to illustrate how manual therapy can be used as part of an integrated approach in treatment of patients with pain and joint dysfunction. My goal is reduction of pain and increase in functional activities. There will always be alternatives on how to reach this goal.

First, I want to restate a few principles of importance when planning the treatment:

— The sequence of normal development is used as one of the guidelines for planning the treatment program.
   This does not mean that the adult patient has to do the same activity as the child, but that the activity the patient does, gives him a similar sensory feedback as the child's activity.
— The joints are considered both as receptors and biomechanical structures.
— The autonomic reactions are taken into account.
— Pain or discomfort should not increase under or after the treatment.
— Increase in range of motion is only a goal if the stability in the new range is adequate.
— Questions like what does the patient need and how much does he tolerate, have to be answered.
— Patient education is an important part of the intervention: what he can do on his own and what must he avoid.
— The patient's age, sex, work habits and leisure-time activities are taken into account when planning the goal of treatment.

In everyday practice, a trial treatment is given after a tentative outline has been made. However, the different procedures chosen are adjusted all the time to the patient's reaction. The treatment process itself, with the afferent feedback it gives the therapist, is the best continuous evaluation tool. The suggested treatment must be practical to the patient and the therapist.

Example 1

The first example, patient A, suffered a fracture of the radius 6 weeks ago and was referred to the therapist after the cast was removed. The patient shows many of the signs mentioned under the evaluation regarding a candidate for reflex sympathetic dystrophy. He carries his arm close to his body; the hand is swollen, painful and hypersensitive to touch. The whole arm bothers him, and he is reluctant to move the arm and hand. When he takes his shirt off, it is evident that he has limited range of motion in his shoulder and hand.

At this stage manual therapy procedures are contraindicated, and would most likely increase pain and give other unwanted reactions.

Other stimuli that must be avoided are:
— extremes of temperature
— placing demands on the patient that he perceives as too great, for example too many home exercises, or exercises that are too difficult or too heavy
— anything that increases the patient's anxiety, for example, lack of information or badly given information

Does the patient, in fact, need information and assurance first?

How can the patient as a whole be influenced so that specific stimuli applied later, such as active movements and joint mobilization, will not produce adverse reactions?

The patient needs to have the activity in his sympathetic nervous system dampened before anything else is attempted.

What are the alternatives for this specific type of patient?

Connective tissue massage (Teirich-Leube, 1978) is hypothesized to have this dampening effect, and this is also my experience. Since the tolerance to any type of stimuli is limited, the dosage is started very low. The details in this treatment approach will not be discussed. Reduction of pain and oedema, together with increased functional activity are signs of improvement and indicators that the treatment can be progressed.

There are other alternatives for dampening the sympathetic tone. According to Rood (Stockmeyer, 1967, 1969) several procedures are hypothesized to have this effect.

Some of these are:
— slow stroking down the posterior primary rami for up to 3 minutes
— slow rhythmical movements of the body, for example in a rocking chair
— neutral warmth
— breathing exercises to encourage relaxed diaphragmatic breathing

The treatment can be progressed with gentle activities to mobilize the shoulder and hand. Joint mobilization as such is still not the choice.

Gentle activites could, for example, be:
— rotation of the body in relation to the arm in sidelying
— sitting with the forearm on the table, rocking back and forth.

These movements are done without producing pain, and the range in flexion and extention in the shoulder joint is adjusted accordingly.

When the patient is able to tolerate slight movements of the hand, he can roll the hand on top of a soft ball. Gentle movements will occur in the wrist, metacarpal and carpal joints. The hand will also get accustomed to touch.

Finally, the patient will be 'ready' for specific joint mobilization procedures. Joint mobilization is performed in the loose-packed position and always started with traction. When traction is used to relieve pain, the pull is only great enough to release the compression effect in the joint or to move the distal joint partner as far as the tissues allow. If there is a pain component, gliding is performed first in the direction of least restriction. When testing joint play the patient may show limitation in one direction, and too much movement in another direction. It is important that the gliding is only done in the restricted direction.

According to Kaltenborn (1980), the distal joint partner is most often moved in relation to the proximal joint partner. Care is taken that the proximal joint partner is stabilized, and straps are used to stabilize the pelvis or the shoulder girdle, or to fasten the patient to the table.

My view on and practice of joint mobilization are influenced by the Rood approach. As mentioned earlier, I am hypersensitive to the patient's autonomic reactions and very reluctant to do procedures that increase the patient's pain. I am alert to the latency effect of the treatment.

When doing joint mobilization I follow the concave–convex rule, but I start mobilizing the *proximal* joint partner in relation to the distal joint partner. Somehow it feels less frightening to have the larger part moved, and the patient is able to relax more and tolerates movements without getting more pain. The perception of the movement is different, and is expressed in terms like, 'it feels more like I am doing it myself'.

The hands of the therapist should be perceived as friendly, making the patient feel secure but not forced as if he is in a straight-jacket. Consequently, I do not use straps. When applying traction to the whole extremity, the pull is never greater than the force needed to release the compression effect in the joint. Normally, this does not have any adverse reaction on the spine. If, however, the patient has had a disc problem not long ago, traction of the extremity would produce asymmetrical pull on the spine and would be contraindicated.

It is my experience that it is crucial to select the right rhythm and amplitude for the individual patient when doing joint mobilization. The gliding movements are performed rhythmically and repeatedly throughout the range or at the end of range, according to the patient's need. The movements get the character of oscillations. Maitland (1977) has described how he uses oscillations both in physiological movements and movements of joint play in order to reduce pain. According to Wyke (1981), stimulation of the mechanoreceptors are one possibility for the reduction of pain.

Joint mobilization as mentioned is started in the small joints of the wrist, hand and fingers, bearing in mind that the patient may regress to the dystrophic stage if treatment and his own activities are overdone.

Mobilization procedures for the shoulder may be relevant, but these are more closely described for the next patient. Finally, the patient needs to use the hand and arm in doing quick or unexpected movements.

The next two examples are from patients with pain and dysfunction in the shoulder joint.

Example 2

Patient B fell on the snow 2 months ago. After the first pain had subsided, he had difficulty in getting his hand into his back-pocket, and it was slightly painful to put on his coat.

The evaluation revealed that he had limited active and passive range of motion in the shoulder joint. The limitation was according to a capsular pattern; joint play was limited in the dorsal and caudal direction. Pain increased at the end of the range, both actively and passively in the same direction. There was also muscle spasm around the joint.

Patient B has both an arthrogenic and neuromuscular problem.

The arthrogenic problem:
Range of motion in his shoulder is less than normal, due to limited gliding of the head of the humerus in dorsal and caudal directions.

When the bone movement is forced beyond the gliding in the joint, the movement axis is shifted to the periphery of the joint as described under instability. When movements are done to the extremes of his range he will have compression on one point together with stretch on the opposite side of the joint. This mostly produces pain.

The neuromuscular problem:
— The rotator cuff is inhibited and has lost much of its function
— The more phasic muscles have taken over the holding functions and become short and hypertonic.
  The goal is to reverse this:
— Facilitate the stabilizing function of the rotator cuff
— Inhibit the more phasic muscles around the shoulder.

This is an excellent example to illustrate how joint mobilization and PNF patterns and techniques can be used together to the patient's benefit. The treatment is started with traction, oscillations and gliding in the painfree range in order to increase joint play. The proximal joint member is the scapula, which is moved first: later the caput humeri is moved in relation to the scapula.

Among the relaxation techniques in PNF there are several alternatives. The technique slow reversal—hold—relax would address the more phasic muscles, but has very little to offer the more tonic muscles.

The technique of choice is most likely rhythmic stabilization— as simultaneous contractions of antagonists. The rotator cuff is facilitated and the more phasic muscles inhibited. The resistance is moderated to the patient's response. The patient is not supposed to push or pull but to maintain the contraction in a co-contraction pattern. This procedure is performed in a part of the range where the roll-gliding in the joint is adequate, in a flexion–abduction or flexion–adduction pattern. In this way joint mobilization and rhythmic stabilization can be used together, the therapist being aware that biomechanical principles and neuromuscular mechanisms have to work together. Therefore, joint play is increased first, muscle function is then retrained for every new degree of movement.

The next step is to instruct the patient to move his body in relation to his extremities, in standing and sitting positions, or hands and knees. The movements are rocking back and forth, or diagonal motion. Rocking back stimulates the appropriate roll-gliding in the joint. The range of motion in these activites stays within the available roll-gliding in the joint, in order to get normal sensory feedback and not produce the unwanted compression in the joint.

Example 3

The last example, patient C, also fell 5 weeks ago. He felt a sharp pain in the shoulder at the time of injury. The shoulder hurt for the first 3 weeks, and the arm was difficult to use.

Evaluation showed that there was limited range of motion in the shoulder, but the active range was more limited than the passive range of motion.

This patient has mainly a neuromuscular problem—with lack of stabilizing functions—the rotator cuff is not stabilizing the head of the humerus during the range of movement. In this case joint mobilization is not indicated, as neuromuscular instability is the main problem.

Pendulum exercises to increase range of motion may be appropriate. Again, rhythmic stabilization techniques to facilitate the rotator cuff in different parts of the range is appropriate, most likely starting in a position where the head of the humerus is in a middle position.

Co-contraction patterns are also done with the distal end fixed in different degrees of flexion in the shoulder joint. Weight bearing is increased and movement is added. All the time the therapist must observe and palpate to make sure the stabilization of the shoulder and scapula is adequate.

Finally, slow reversal techniques through the range could be used to teach normal timing through alternating movements.

SUMMARY

I have purposely taken all the examples from the upper extremity in order to illustrate how manual therapy can be used together with other treatment approaches in order to treat pain and joint dysfunction. The same principles of evaluation and treatment as described here can be adapted to any part of the body when the goal is to reduce pain and restore function. Pain is regarded as a symptom. Treating pain without evaluating possible causes is a symptomatic treatment that quite often will not prevent the recurrence of pain and dysfunction, as well as hide the real cause of pain and dysfunction.

REFERENCES

Cookson F 1979 Orthopedic manual therapy—an overview Part II: The spine. Physical Therapy 59: 259–267

Cookson F, Kent B 1979 Orthopedic manual therapy—an overview Part I: The Extremities. Physical Therapy 59: 136–146

Cyriax J H 1975 Textbook of orthopaedic medicine, vol. I Diagnosis of soft tissue lesions, 6th edn. Williams and Wilkins, Baltimore

Ellingsen R-R 1981 Integration of therapeutic methods for evaluation and treatment of motor disorders. Massachusetts General Hospital, unpublished notes

Freeman M A R 1965 Coordination exercises in the treatment of the functional instability of the foot. Physiotherapy 51: 393–395

Freeman M A R et al 1965 The etiology and prevention of functional instability of the foot. The Journal of Bone and Joint Surgery 47B: 678–685

Heiniger M C, Randolph S L 1981 Neurophysiological concepts in human behavior, The tree of learning. The C.V. Mosby Company, St. Louis

Kaltenborn F M 1980 Mobilization of the extremity joints, 3rd edn. Olaf Norlis Bokhandel, Oslo

Knott M, Voss D 1968 Proprioceptive neuromuscular facilitation: Patterns and techniques, 2nd edn. Harper and Row, New York

Maitland G D 1977 Peripheral manipulation, 2nd edn. Butterworths, London

Polly H F, Hunder G G 1978 Rheumatologic interviewing and physical examination of the joints, 2nd edn. W.B Saunders Company, London

Semans S, 1967 The Bobath concept in treatment of neurological disorders. American Journal of Physical Medicine 46: 732–785

Stockmeyer S A 1967 An interpretation of the approach of Rood to the treatment of neuromuscular dysfunction. American Journal of Physical Medicine 46: 900–961

Stockmeyer S A 1969 Course notes

Teirich-Leube H 1978 Grundriss der Bindegewebsmassage. 8 Auflage Gustav Fischer Verlag; Stuttgart

Williams P L, Warwick R 1980 Gray's anatomy 36th edn. Longman, London

Wyke B 1981 The neurology of joints: a review of general principles. Clinics in Rheumatic Diseases vol 7, no 1. W B Saunders Company, London, pp 223–239

Electromyographic feedback and the painful hemiplegic shoulder

INTRODUCTION

Cerebrovascular disease, or stroke, constitutes a major problem in our Western society. It has been estimated that the mortality among stroke patients is about a third and that a reasonable recovery may be expected of a third more. The remaining third who survive, however, will have a moderate to severe handicap, posing problems for themselves, their immediate families or for those who care for them (Evans, 1981).

A unilateral cerebrovascular lesion will produce a symptom complex known as hemiplegia: a paralysis of limbs, trunk, and lower face of the contralateral side. As a result, the motor deficit, involving weakness and spasticity, is found to contribute to the hemiplegic posture. Other disabilities which are not diagnosed so readily, may involve sensation, perception, vision or communication, all of which provide a formidable challenge for those in close association with the hemiplegic patient.

Various secondary complications following stroke may occur because of underlying medical problems, age and perhaps inadequate or ineffective care. Of particular interest to physical therapists at this time are the problems of spasticity and pain in the shoulder.

Following the initial flaccid phase, developing spasticity, the presence of abnormal reflex activity, sensory impairment and perceptual deficits usually prevent movement of the shoulder. In particular, movements against gravity are found to be difficult or impossible. Inactivity of the shoulder and arm will then lead to later problems of the upper extremity. Clinically, one such problem is pain (Moskowitz, 1969; Inabe & Piorkowski, 1972; Cailliet, 1980; Jensen, 1980). This may be located at the shoulder and become more intense during motion of the arm, or it may be a continuous pain which radiates to the arm and hand, interrupting sleep and remaining unaffected by analgesics or physical therapy. The primary pain often continues for an indefinite period of time leading

183

to a frozen shoulder and later is consistent with the complex symptom of post-traumatic reflex sympathetic dystrophy (Najenson & Pikielny, 1965; Moskowitz, 1969; Inaba & Piorkowski, 1972; Kozin et al, 1976; Davis et al, 1977; Johnstone, 1978; Cailliet, 1980; Jensen, 1980). Cailliet (1980) indicated that the painful hemiplegic shoulder will often result in the five D's: disuse atrophy, disability, depression, drugs and dependence.

A file search for all hemiplegic patients admitted to a rehabilitation centre in Quebec between January 1976 and March 1979, revealed that of 445 patients admitted during this three year period, 157 (37%) demonstrated shoulder pain in association with spasticity (Williams, 1980). These 157 patients first complained of pain anywhere between 3 and 16 weeks post stroke. Before discussing further the possible causes of shoulder pain in the hemiplegic patient, some relevant facts concerning the anatomy and function of the normal joint should perhaps be considered.

Scapulohumeral movement

For every 15° of abduction of the arm, 10° occur at the glenohumeral joint, and 5° from rotation of the scapula upon the chest wall. This two to one ratio of the humerus to the scapula exists throughout the entire range of abduction. This smooth integrated movement of the shoulder complex has been well termed 'scapulohumeral rhythm' (Codman, 1934). Without scapular rotation, the humerus therefore cannot fully abduct or elevate overhead (Cailliet, 1978). This is often found to be the situation among the hemiplegic patients (Basmajian, 1967; Johnstone, 1978; Jensen, 1980).

Scapulohumeral movement in hemiplegia

In hemiplegia the muscles that permit the aforementioned scapulohumeral rhythm are impaired, firstly by flaccidity of the surrounding musculature and later by developing spasticity in the antagonistic muscles, particularly the shoulder depressor muscles: pectoralis major, latissimus dorsi, teres major and minor and infraspinatus, biceps and coracobrachialis (Brunnstrom, 1970; Bobath, 1978; Johnstone, 1978).

The inferior angle of the scapula is also fixed by the action of the spastic rhomboid and trapezius muscles. It is therefore prevented from moving outwards and upwards with elevation of the arm. If the arm is passively forced upwards, the necessary rotation of the scapula and elevation of the acromion do not take place. As a result, the humerus is pressed against the acromion and the patient will complain of pain (Voss, 1967; Bryce et al, 1977; Bobath, 1978; Johnstone, 1978; Cailliet, 1980).

It becomes apparent that the hemiplegic patients' problem is not one concerning paralysis of certain muscles. It is rather an inhibition of certain muscle groups caused by the powerful spastic contraction of other muscle groups. One important large muscle among the strong group of depressor muscles of the shoulder is the latissimus dorsi. The major action of this muscle is to retract and depress the shoulder. Clinically, the stroke patient is invariably found to exhibit strong spasticity within this muscle. Because of the size and origins of this large hypertonic muscle there will also be lateral trunk shortening on the stroke patients' affected side (Johnstone, 1978; Cailliet, 1978).

Possible causes of the painful hemiplegic shoulder

In many instances, the flaccid and hypotonic hanging arm will subluxate due to the lack of normal muscle and ligamentous support necessary to maintain articulation of the head of the humerus with the glenoid cavity of the scapula (Cailliet, 1980; Chino, 1981). Subluxation may also occur as a result of the changed slope of the glenoid cavity, when the normal locking mechanism of abduction is prevented (Basmajian, 1967; Fitzgerald & Gibson, 1975; Jensen, 1980). Subluxation may be noted early at the flail shoulder, or with the ensuing signs of spasticity, or it may later complicate the chronic severe spastic extremity (Johnstone, 1978).

The function of the supraspinatus muscle, and the significance of this muscle in subluxation of the glenohumeral joint in hemiplegia, was investigated by Chaco and Wolf (1971). They demonstrated that loading on the shoulder joint should be avoided while the affected limb is in the flaccid state, in order to prevent subluxation. Others have shown, both morphologically and electromyographically, that subluxation is possible following the forced movement of shoulder abduction (Basmajian, 1967; Chino, 1981).

Cailliet (1980) emphasized that it is important to decide whether the cause of subluxation at the shoulder is that of paralysis of the supporting muscles or a lesion of the articular capsule. In other words, is it likely to be a permanent condition or will the subluxation diminish as muscle tone is restored? As indicated by Jensen (1980), however, a study of this question is difficult to perform in hemiplegic patients as they demonstrate such variations of muscle tone, severity of paresis and recovery period. Certain authors cite the coracohumeral ligament, in particular, as a prime source of dysfunction (Cailliet, 1980; Jensen, 1980).

In the normal shoulder the coracohumeral ligament functions as a braking mechanism for shoulder motion, especially when the arm is moved to extreme positions (Johnston & Willis, 1973). If this ligament is injured, the shoulder loses its braking mechanism, allowing the rotator cuff muscles to be over-stretched. This may result in an inferior subluxation of the humeral head through the effect of gravity on the arm (Najenson et al, 1971; de Bats et al, 1974; Fitzgerald & Gibson, 1975; Cailliet, 1978).

Degenerative changes in the articular capsule, seen normally with progressing age, are found to be the most pronounced at the site of the coracohumeral ligament (Olsson, 1953). The elderly hemiplegic patient is likely, therefore, to have degenerative changes prior to the onset of stroke. Without the protective mechanism of the shoulder muscles these patients are particularly vulnerable toward injury of the coracohumeral ligament (Cailliet, 1980). Also of consequence, and effecting stroke cases of all ages, is the fact that the voluntarily controlled rotation of the humerus has been eliminated due to the paretic rotator cuff. If the arm is passively abducted past 90%, the required rotation will happen forcibly; the greater tuberosity of the humerus will press against the acromion with possible danger of damage to interjacent soft tissue (Basmajian, 1967; Bobath, 1978; Cailliet, 1980; Jensen, 1980).

By the use of plain shoulder x-rays and shoulder arthrographies, Najenson et al (1971) found that 40% of patients with an effected hemiplegic shoulder suffered concomitantly from rupture of the rotator cuff. This was accompanied in all cases by severe pain in the glenohumeral joint and tenderness on pressure of the greater tuberosity of the humerus. Nepomuceno and Miller (1974) also made use of contrast arthrography in a study which included 24 hemiplegic patients with painful and/or stiff shoulder joints. All patients denied premorbid pathology. Seven (33%) demonstrated a rotator cuff tear and one had a transverse bicipital tendon tear. Five of the eight with abnormal arthrograms showed clinical subluxation. The authors were uncertain whether these lesions were spontaneous or due to secondary complications. They indicated that trauma may have been overlooked at the time of the stroke. On the other hand, they suspected that this type of injury is more likely to occur while patients are performing activities of daily living (ADL) in the ward, or later when at home.

Other later complications of the hemiplegic shoulder likely to cause pain and dysfunction are frozen shoulder, an impairment of the hand-arm-shoulder venous lymphatic circulation known as shoulder-hand-finger syndrome, or a reflex sympathetic dystrophy syndrome (Moskowitz, 1969; Kozin et al, 1976; Davis et al, 1977; Jensen, 1980; Marduel, 1980). The fact that the hemiplegic patient with a flail arm cannot actively elevate, forward flex or abduct the arm in order to place the hand in a functional anti-gravity position is of undoubted significance. The time between the onset of stroke and the first symptoms of shoulder-hand-finger syndrome has been estimated by Davis et al (1977). They showed that most patients developed symptoms and signs between the second and third month after the onset of hemiplegia.

One of the factors often cited as a cause of the painful shoulder in the hemiplegic patient is inappropriate handling and positioning of the involved extremity (Najenson et al, 1971). Different groups of workers in hospitals carry out procedures which may harm the paretic shoulder. Jensen (1980) stated that the pain is often due to a 'too strenuous and ignorant manipulation of a joint lacking physiological function'.

One cause of an immobile scapula is spasticity of the shoulder retractors. As already mentioned, the typical distribution of spasticity seen in hemiplegia may well include the retractors and depressor muscles of the shoulder (Todd, 1974; Bryce et al, 1977; Bobath, 1978; Johnstone, 1978).

A further cause of pain that warrants consideration may be that of sensory deprivation. Melzack (1973) proposed that chronic pathological pain may lead to permanent or semi-permanent changes in the central nervous system (CNS). These changes could be in the form of self-exciting neuron chains (Jeans, 1978). Melzack and Casey (1968) suggested that the drive mechanisms associated with pain are activated when the somato-sensory input exceeds a critical level. More information is needed, however, before this last cause can be linked with hemiplegic shoulder pain.

The literature would indicate, therefore, that pain of the shoulder and arm in the hemiplegic patient may arise from malalignment and subluxation of the glenohumeral joint, possible rupture of the coracohumeral ligament or rotator cuff muscles, frozen shoulder or, later, shoulder-hand-finger syndrome or possible sensory deprivation. The problem may be complicated by the presence of spasticity combined with unskilled and often strenuous treatment of a joint. Functionally, recovery of the stroke patient can therefore be greatly impeded by the often persistent pain at the shoulder (Johnstone, 1978).

Little attention has been given in the literature to the treatment of pain associated with spasticity at the hemiplegic shoulder. A few authors have, however, suggested that relaxation of the strong shoulder depressor muscles could later increase the movement of the hemiplegic shoulder (Bobath, 1978; Johnstone, 1978; Cailliet, 1980). As previously mentioned, pain is associated with limitation, if not total prevention, of movement.

It can be hypothesized, therefore, that by reducing spasticity at the shoulder, especially of the shoulder depressor muscles, range of movement could possibly be increased. This could provide an influx of arterial blood to all the tissues surrounding the joint (Nouwen & Solinger, 1979), which in turn might help alleviate the pain.

Rationale for study of relaxation of involved muscles

In hemiplegic patients, there is no reciprocal relaxation of the antagonists by contraction of the agonists (Brunnstrom, 1970; Bobath, 1978; Cailliet, 1980). A direct approach towards relaxation of the spastic antagonists, therefore, is necessary in order to release the prime movers (Cailliet, 1980). One modality in current use for relaxation of spasticity is electromyographic (EMG) biofeedback (Amato et al, 1973; Johnson & Garton, 1973; Swaan et al, 1974; Brudny et al, 1976; Baker et al, 1977; Wolf, 1978; Kelly et al, 1979). Another long-used approach for gaining relaxation that may also be considered, is the application of the Jacobson's Relaxation Method (Jacobson, 1929).

Electromyographic biofeedback as a means to relaxation

Biofeedback is based on the premise that an individual can modify or gain control over a range of bodily functions once thought to be totally automatic. It is essentially a self-educational technique employing electronic information feedback devices. With such equipment, patients can learn how to regulate their own physical and mental processes. This may involve control over muscle activity or the so called 'involuntary' body processes such as blood pressure, body temperature or heart rate. Electromyographic (EMG) biofeedback has been well defined by Green and Green (1975) who stated that 'it is the monitoring of physiological parameters to provide continuous information which is immediately available as a feedback signal in the form of a tone, a light or the movement of a needle on a meter'.

The idea of providing informational feedback related to changes in muscle activity is generally attributed to Marinacci and Horande (1960). They used the clinical electromyograph which is usually employed to determine peripheral nerve conduction velocities and to examine the characteristics of muscle action potentials. By setting the device to monitor raw muscle activity and by listening to the sounds emitted concurrently through an audio amplifier, the first form of visual and auditory feedback of muscle behaviour was provided.

The major application of EMG biofeedback has been in the rehabilitation of stroke patients, with a particular focus on the development of improved ankle dorsiflexion and gait. The outcome from this application has been mixed, as shown in studies by Harrison and Connolly (1971), Johnson and Garton (1973), Amato et al (1973), Burnside et al (1979). Nonetheless, these investigators demonstrated that EMG biofeedback training may be effective in achieving functional activity when other therapies have failed.

Information is available in the literature on the role of EMG biofeedback and its use in achieving relaxation of spastic musculature. More specifically, evidence has implicated EMG biofeedback training as a valuable technique in assisting patients who have had a stroke, especially when trying to regain functional control over spastic musculature (Basmajian et al, 1975; Brudny et al, 1976; Kelly et al, 1979; Wolf et al, 1980).

One such study designed to investigate the use of EMG in hypertonic subjects monitored the level of activity in the spastic forearm flexor muscles (Harrison & Connolly, 1971). The results showed that the level of control attained by the four hypertonic patients was as fine as that achieved by the four normal subjects. The abnormal subjects, however, took appreciably longer to gain this control. Details concerning the application of the biofeedback are lacking and the two groups were very small.

A later study by Brudny et al (1976) reviewed 35 hemiplegic patients who had received biofeedback training for the upper extremity three times a week for a period of 8–12 weeks. Involvement of the upper extremity was graded on a 4 point scale. Four patients showed no change, 4 relief of spasticity only, and 27 demonstrated improved functional ability. This study did not take into account the baseline characteristics. The reader, therefore, cannot appreciate the before and after treatment situation in order to make any comparisons.

Wolf et al (1979) used a biofeedback training regime which required a reduction of amplitude and frequency of recorded EMG in hypertonic muscles. They also noted the time required to regain resting EMG activity after first slow and then rapid, manual stretching. Of 32 patients with upper and lower limb involvement, 18 lower extremities were tested successfully while only 5 upper extremities achieved comparable results. A reason for this difference may be that a limb which showed an improvement in shoulder and elbow mobility but failed to achieve functional prehension, was not rated as a successful outcome.

Among the studies reviewed, there appears to be a consensus of opinion that biofeedback training enables some patients, particularly those whose performance had previously plateaued, to gain a degree of control of hypertonic muscle groups and increased contraction in paretic groups. It is only on the rare occasion, however, that one can read of any specific details in regard to placement of electrodes, position of patient or length of biofeedback sessions.

Similarly, there are few studies that determine the effect of patient characteristics on outcome. One such study by Wolf et al (1979), however, suggests that the age, sex, hemiparetic side, duration of previous rehabilitation and number of biofeedback training sessions are not significantly related to treatment outcomes. They indicated that the presence of aphasia reduces the prospects for a successful outcome and proprioceptive deficits seem to be a major obstacle to achieving improved limb function.

All the preceding studies reviewed on EMG biofeedback required the patient to understand and carry out instructions and to also be reasonably well motivated in order to follow through on the training program. Many of the patients had reached a plateau of recovery using conventional treatment methods. Subjects often acted as their own control, and thus any improvement was perhaps attributable to biofeedback training rather than natural recovery processes. All training programs were structured so that spasticity was first reduced in the resting position, then under conditions of increasing difficulty. Sensitivity of the biofeedback amplifier was correspondingly altered from the easiest to the most difficult settings, by use of the threshold selector. The number of treatments given in these studies varied widely. As pointed out by Grynbaum et al (1976) patients may respond very rapidly or require months of treatment.

Jacobson's relaxation method

This procedure, known also as progressive relaxation, emphasizes that people can learn proprioceptive awareness of tension and then use it in almost any situation to relax from a state of tension. Following this approach, habit patterns tend to develop, with a resultant increase in the ability to relax voluntarily (Jacobson, 1929).

Relaxation is taught in a quiet semidarkened room, with the patient comfortably positioned and all parts of the body well supported. Constricting garments should be loosened. Prolonged slow breathing with proper diaphragmatic and abdominal coordination, together with intercostal breathing, is taught, thereby gaining good breath control. The patient is reminded to exhale slowly through the mouth to emphasize awareness of the breathing rate.

In order to learn how to relax, the subject must first learn how a static contraction or tenseness feels and attempt to release this contraction. Each group of muscles is taken in turn and the larger groups are usually concentrated on first. Proprioceptive awareness is, therefore, enhanced as the patient feels the difference between tightness and relaxation of the contracting muscles. Following a strong voluntary contraction, the patient is asked to relax. Then progressively weaker contractions are alternated with complete inhibition of muscular activity so that the part becomes fully relaxed. As the patient becomes aware of the sensations associated with a muscular contraction, he becomes able to initiate or inhibit that contraction (Jacobson, 1929).

By the use of electromyography and cutaneous or intramuscular electrodes, the various involved muscle groups can be monitored. This will in turn indicate to the therapist to what extent relaxation has really been obtained.

RESEARCH STUDY

While earlier studies with hemiplegic patients noted that EMG biofeedback reduced spasticity in the affected lower extremity, little attention has been given to the effect of biofeedback on the painful hemiplegic shoulder. The following study, therefore, sets out to examine the effects of biofeedback, in the early stages of hemiplegia, on pain and range of movement in the involved upper extremity.

Purpose and hypothesis

The purpose of this randomized controlled study (Williams, 1982) was to assess the effect of EMG biofeedback applied to hemiplegic patients who had suffered onset of shoulder pain between 3 and 16 weeks post-stroke. It was hypothesized that by encouraging relaxation, pain and spasticity might be reduced, thus increasing the range of movement at the shoulder.

Method

The study was conducted at a 120 bed urban rehabilitation hospital* where patients requiring intensive rehabilitation are treated as inpatients. Twenty right-handed subjects, 11 males and 9 females, were included in the simple, their age ranging from 37 years to 81 years with a mean age of 63.5 years (SD = 11.8). Patients were selected according to the following criteria; each must (a) have a diagnosis of hemiplegia or hemiparesis secondary to vascular disease (thrombosis, embolism); (b) be between 3 and 16 weeks post-stroke; (c) have a painful shoulder on the hemiplegic side; (d) have no previous history of shoulder pain prior to stroke; (e) have the ability to follow instructions and not show any signs of receptive aphasia; (f) not be receiving any medication to reduce spasticity; (g) be able to understand English or French; (h) have signed an informed consent form, or a responsible individual have signed on his behalf.

Patients meeting these criteria were initially screened, interviewed and assessed for motor function and sensation by the study director. The scoring system used was adapted from the Fugl-Meyer et al (1975) classification of motor recovery following stroke. This provided a means of 'staging' patients for possible prognosis; for instance, patients in Stage I or II were considered to be in a 'poor' category and those in Stages III to V in a 'good' category. During a stratification process, these two categories were later found to be evenly distributed between the two groups, each having 6 patients with a poor prognosis and 4 with a good prognosis.

Case histories showed that these were the first strokes for all subjects (mean time since onset of stroke for the sample was 7 weeks). Twelve subjects had left-sided involvement and 8 right-sided in-

*Jewish Convalescent Hospital, 3805 Alton Goldbloom, Chomedey, Laval, Quebec

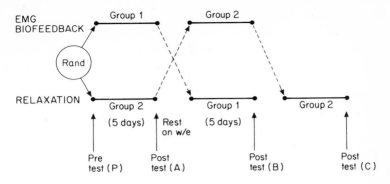

Fig. 8.1 Diagram of cross-over design.

volvement. These subjects were also found to be evenly distributed between the two groups.

Experimental design

A cross-over design was employed (Fig. 8.1) with each patient acting as his own control. After screening, each patient was randomly assigned to either Group 1 or 2 and then assessed by the 'blind' evaluator. Those in group 1 received EMG biofeedback for a half-hour period on 5 consecutive days (B-R). Patients in Group 2 received instruction in general relaxation for a half-hour period on 2 consecutive days (R-B). All patients were simultaneously undergoing conventional physical therapy.

At the end of week one, all subjects were reassessed by the 'blind' evaluator and reassigned to the opposite treatment group. The treatment protocols were then repeated, and subjects were again re-evaluated at the end of week two. Those patients receiving biofeedback during week two were reassessed at the end of week three as a follow-up to the EMG biofeedback treatment.

Treatment procedures

The conventional physical therapy program for all patients lasted one hour. It had nothing to do with the study and was given by various therapists within the physical therapy department, where consistent use is made of the neurodevelopment approach to treatment (Bobath, 1978).

During the study, each patient received their treatment sessions in the sitting position with the involved upper extremity supported on a pillow. In order to aid relaxation, a reflex-inhibiting pattern (RIP) was encouraged.

Each relaxation session lasted 30 minutes and was taught by the study director. The technique followed was that of the Jacobson method of relaxation (Jacobson, 1929). During the initial week, Group 2 (R-B) was the group given the relaxation. Group 1 (B-R), however, was also given instruction in relaxation in conjunction with the first two EMG biofeedback treatments.

The EMG biofeedback was provided by the Autogen 1700 machine*. This machine has a logarithmic meter for visual display, an audiofeedback with seven audiofeedback modes, and a light feedback. The meter provides instantaneous or time-averaged EMG readouts with a ten-turn feedback threshold selector. The use and operation of the machine was carefully explained to the patient and a short demonstration given on the patient's unaffected side. Following careful skin preparation, two surface electrodes (Standard Beckman)** were placed over the upper tendinous area of latissimus dorsi and teres major. A suitable electrode site was predetermined by asking the patient to raise the *unaffected* arm and then adduct and inwardly rotate it against resistance. It was then possible to palpate the upper tendinous area of latissimus dorsi on the posterior aspect of the shoulder. A similar placement site could then be selected on the affected side.

A recording of the sensitivity level of the integrated EMG at rest was made both at the beginning and end of each session and its significance explained to the patient. It was then understood that by relaxing, the subject could reduce the noise level of the biofeedback machine and lower the meter reading, thereby decreasing the electrical activity of the muscles being monitored.

Each patient received 5 (daily) treatments of the EMG biofeedback lasting between 20 and 25 minutes per session, excluding preparation of the skin, the relaxation period and time spent in giving instructions to the patient. The aim throughout was to obtain relaxation of the two shoulder depressor muscles being monitored, namely latissimus dorsi and teres major muscles.

Evaluation procedures

Two dependent variables, pain and range of movement, were eval-

* Autogen Systems, Inc., 809 Allston Way, Berkeley, California, 94710, U.S.A.

** Beckman Instruments, Inc., 3900 River Road, Schiller Park, Illinois, 60176, U.S.A.

uated by a physical therapist who was unaware of the purpose of this trial and had no responsibility for the conventional treatment of the subjects. She was taught specific training procedures in order to provide a uniform approach towards the evaluation of all involved patients, thus reducing the possibility of bias.

Two instruments were used in the study to measure the dependent variables. The McGill Pain Questionnaire, Part I to IV (Melzack, 1975) was used to measure pain, and a gravity reference electro-goniometer[†] was used to record the range of movement of the affected shoulder (Peat & Grahame, 1976).

1. The McGill Pain Questionnaire, which has been validated and shown to be reliable (Melzack, 1975), provided quantitative information concerning the location, type and severity of pain experienced by the patient in the involved shoulder. There are three measures in the index but only two were used in the study. One,

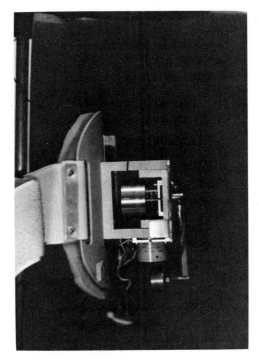

Fig. 8.2 Electrogoniometer to measure range of movement at the shoulder joint.

† Developed by Dr M. Peat, School of Physical Therapy, University of Western Ontario, London, Ontario, Canada

the Pain Rating Index (PRI), is based on ranked values of words chosen by the patient to describe the pain, giving, therefore, a total number which could be recorded at every evaluation. The second, the Present Pain Intensity Scale (PPI), ranks the degree of pain from mild to excruciating. These pain levels were recorded daily on a separate index card for each patient.

2. *The gravity reference electrogoniometer* (Peat & Grahame, 1976), together with a 419A DC null voltmeter*, provided a method of recording two single-plane passive arm movements, namely, flexion and abduction (Fig. 8.2). Prior to the study, the electrogoniometer and voltmeter had been inspected for electromechanical integrity, and duly calibrated.

Results

Although there were no significant differences found in the outcome scores between the two groups after week one or week two, the

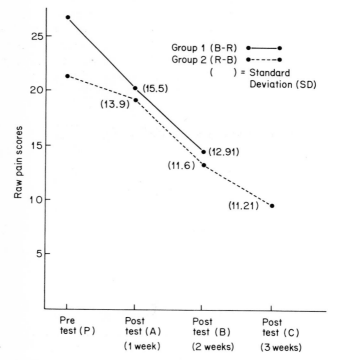

Fig. 8.3 Comparison of mean pain scores between groups over the study period.

* Hewlet-Packard, Loveland Instrument Division, P.O. 301, Loveland, Colorado, 80537, USA.

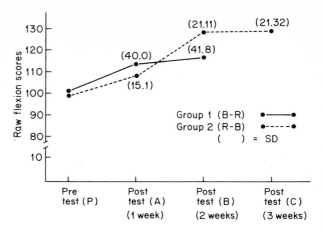

Fig. 8.4 Comparison of mean range of flexion scores between groups over the study period.

mean scores did demonstrate a trend in improvement (Figs. 8.3, 8.4, 8.5). Both groups when tested within groups after week one or week two did, however, show a significant decrease in pain. Furthermore, Group 2 (R-B) also showed a significant decrease in pain and increase in range of movement at the end of week two.

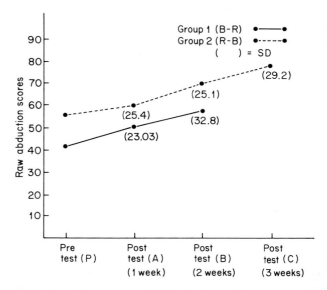

Fig. 8.5 Comparison of mean range of abduction-scores between groups over the study period.

Analysis

The validity and reliability of the equipment was tested by means of a Pearson product-moment correlation. The recordings were highly correlated (r = 0.99). Moreover, an intra-therapist reliability study also indicated that the evaluator's recordings were reliable (r = 0.75).

By means of t-tests, initial patient characteristics, such as time since onset of stroke, age, the initial motor function, sensation, pain and range of movement, were analyzed to determine if the randomization had been successful in creating two well-balanced groups. No significant differences were found at the probability level of 0.05. Other characteristics, which included diagnosis, side of involvement and prognostic category, were compared by the use of a chi-square distribution. Again, there were no significant differences at the probability level of 0.05.

The specific shoulder problems were also considered. It was found that Group 1 (B-R) had 7 subjects with a subluxated shoulder (4 right-sided and 3 left-sided), while Group 2 (R-B) had 6 subjects with subluxated shoulder (2 right-sided and 4 left-sided). Each group had one subject with a shoulder-hand syndrome only, and one with capsulitis only. Group 1 (B-R) had 1 subject with a rotator-cuff injury, whereas Group 2 (R-B) had 2 with a frozen shoulder. When comparing shoulder subluxation versus any other named shoulder problem between the two groups, the chi-square distribution showed no difference at the 0.05 level.

For the study itself, the assumed null hypothesis was that there would be no differences between the effect of EMG biofeedback and that of relaxation. A test of significance, a series of two tailed t-tests, was applied to compare the pain scores and range of movement scores, between groups.

Furthermore, by use of the cross-over design, the pain scores and the mean range of movement scores from week one and week two were compared within groups. Paired t-tests were used for this purpose.

There was a further week of follow-up (without training) for Group 2 (R-B), in order to test for any carry-over effects from the EMG biofeedback. The same variables as above were, therefore, again tested by means of a paired t-test. The level of significance for all statistical analysis was set at 0.05. The records kept by the study director provided additional descriptive data from the daily pain record cards and from the EMG biofeedback treatment logs. The average decrease in EMG activity for each patient during the five biofeedback sessions was recorded.

At the end of week one, the comparison of treatment outcomes with regard to the variables, pain, range of movement and percentage of movement scores, showed that although there were differences between the two groups they were not statistically significant at the 0.05 level. However, as seen in Figures 8.3, 8.4, and 8.5, the mean levels did show a trend of improvement, with Group 1 (B-R) demonstrating a greater decrease in pain and more improvement in range of movement than group 2 (R-B).

The differences between the two groups analyzed in terms of such variables as motor function, sensation, pain, range of movement and percentage of movement scores at the end of week two, again showed differences which were not statistically significant at the 0.05 level. Once more, however, the mean improvement levels did show a trend, with Group 2 (R-B) demonstrating a greater improvement in range of movement than Group 1 (B-R) (Figs. 8.4 and 8.5). At this time, the decrease in pain was found to be approximately the same for both groups (Fig. 8.3).

A significant improvement of pain scores for both groups was found within groups after two weeks. Group 2 (R-B) also showed a significant improvement in range of movement of flexion and abduction.

Furthermore, the comparison of variables within Group 2 (R-B) at the end of week two and three, showed significant improvement with regard to pain scores ($p = 0.013$). A trend of improvement in range of movement was also noted.

Descriptive information

As already mentioned, the descriptive data obtained included pain record scores and the EMG biofeedback treatment log recordings. In Group 1 (B-R), no further pain was reported by 3 patients after week one and by 2 patients after week two; the remaining 5 patients reported a decrease in pain. All patients in Group 2 (R-B) continued to complain of pain after week one, but 6 reported no further pain at the end of week two. Data from both groups indicated that those with a decrease in pain, or no further pain, had reported a better sleep pattern.

A decrease in EMG activity was demonstrated by all patients, the average decrease per session being 1.5 microvolts. The time taken to obtain this decrease, however, varied considerably, ranging anywhere from 5 to 25 minutes per treatment session.

Discussion

The findings from the described study suggest that EMG biofeedback may be effective in the treatment of a painful hemiplegic shoulder. Furthermore, the results obtained may indicate that stroke patients who find it extremely hard to relax, need to learn about relaxation and to lose any fears they may have about the biofeedback machine prior to the treatment procedure.

All subjects, except one in Group 2 (R-B), showed a decrease in pain. For Group 1 (B-R) subjects, the decrease was evenly distributed over the study period, whereas for Group 2 (R-B) the decrease was more marked at the end of week two, after the biofeedback. Pain continued to decrease during week three, suggesting a possible carry-over effect from the biofeedback.

There was a greater increase in passive range of flexion after biofeedback treatments than after the relaxation techniques demonstrated by all subjects. The increase in abduction, however, was not so pronounced. This result was perhaps to be expected as many hemiplegic shoulder problems have been reported to occur following forced abduction (Basmajian, 1967; Chaco & Wolf, 1971; Jensen, 1980). The evaluator always, therefore, took great care to move the limb only within the limit of pain.

As suggested by Wolf et al (1979), many patient characteristics, such as age, sex, hemiparetic side, time interval since the onset of stroke and the number of biofeedback training sessions, may not be significantly related to the treatment outcome. This may apply equally well in the above study to 'prognostic category' obtained from stages of motor recovery. The improvements, noted in both groups, were distributed fairly evenly between 'good' and 'poor' prognostic categories. The small sample population does not, however, allow for any definite statements in terms of prognostic category and treatment outcomes. Perhaps of more importance, when determining possible outcomes, are the level of comprehension and the degree of sensory and proprioceptive impairment.

As noted previously in the literature review, Wolf et al (1979) found that the presence of aphasia and proprioceptive impairment had an impact upon negative outcome. This was more apparent with respect to the lack of improvement in upper rather than lower extremities. There were 4 expressive aphasic patients included in the above study, 2 in each group. All 4 demonstrated a decrease in pain after the biofeedback treatment, but only one in Group 2 (R-B) showed a marked increase in range of movement (flexion, 115° to 140°).

Similarly, patients with low scores in sensation, which included a test for proprioception, tended to do less well than those with high scores. In accordance with Wolf et al (1979), Hurrell (1980) and Walker and Cole (1980), patients with sensory deficits would seem, therefore, to have more difficulty processing information supplied by the EMG biofeedback. This may not necessarily mean that these patients are unsuitable candidates for EMG biofeedback treatment. The processing of sensory information may be distorted. Clinical experience suggests that more time is needed for such patients demonstrating sensory deficits, in order for them to benefit from this modality. Moreover, it may indicate that the application required modification, particularly in reference to the placement of electrodes. Other placement sites could perhaps be chosen where sensation is known to be within normal limits.

The rate at which the subjects in the described study learned to relax varied considerably. Similarly, Grynbaum et al (1976) noted that some patients may respond rapidly, or others may require months of treatment before relaxation is obtained. They did not, however, give specific reasons for this variation. It may well point to a combination of factors; the severity of the cerebral lesion and hence the degree of sensory impairment, are major points for consideration.

As previously mentioned, the use of the cross-over design enabled subjects to act as their own control. Therefore, any improvement could more likely be attributed to the biofeedback training, rather than natural recovery processes. However, as suggested by Hurd et al (1980), results showing improvement may indicate that the effectiveness of this treatment is not necessarily dependent on the exact feedback of myoelectric signals to the patient, but possibly on some other aspect of the treatment design, as yet undefined. Furthermore, Santee et al (1980) pointed out that the role of patient motivation has received little attention in the study of EMG biofeedback programs so far. They indicated that this factor may well have an influence on the outcome.

Several points make this present study somewhat inconclusive and, therefore, it can only be accepted as a pilot study. A different design using a larger sample and possibly a longer period of treatment, together with an extended follow-up period for all patients, would help to further substantiate the outlined result.

The cross-over design was used as the population was small and so allowed for an analysis of data within groups, as well as between groups. It does, however, present disadvantages, especially in terms of the cumulative effect between the different types of treatment intervention. As in this study, Group 2 (R-B) probably had some benefit from the relaxation techniques which in turn could have influenced the EMG biofeedback sessions.

From the literature review, it became evident that the etiology of the painful shoulder remains obscure. The seldom mentioned problem of sensory deprivation may also play a much larger role than has been described in the literature, particularly in reference to the adult hemiplegic. The sensory and proprioceptive stimulation normally received from movement of the upper extremity will be considerably reduced during both the flaccid and spastic phases following a stroke. This may, in turn, cause a distortion of sensory input at the central level. The question then arises as to whether or not this could have anything to do with the interpretation of pain by the hemiplegic patient.

As indicated by Melzack (1973), in some cases of sensory deprivation the normal pattern of impulses received by the CNS may be disorganized or the frequency of impulses excessive. The patient may then experience distorted sensations of pain. The degree of threshold to pain will vary according to the emotional state of the patient. Furthermore, Zimmermann (1979) has suggested that certain states of pain may be due to denervation supersensitivity, sprouting of aberrant nerve connections, or unmasking of ineffective synapses.

Despite the considerable amount of research that has been carried out over the past decade, the key mechanisms of chronic pain are still poorly understood. Therefore, only by further studies concerning chronic pain and more accurate reliable forms of testing sensation and proprioception on the part of the therapist, will the possible role of sensory deprivation, in hemiplegic shoulder pain, become evident. On the other hand, the variation in spasticity during activity is clearly demonstrated in the clinical situation. Accordingly, this present study has shown that relaxation, by the use of EMG biofeedback, may aid reduction of pain and spasticity thus allowing an increase in movement.

CLINICAL IMPLICATIONS OF THE STUDY

The previously described study may indicate that the better order for the two interventions used, is that of relaxation sessions followed by the EMG biofeedback treatment. It is not clearly evident from the results obtained, however, that EMG biofeedback as a form of treatment on its own is of benefit. Rather, it suggests that clinically, when using EMG biofeedback, the physical therapist should first make sure the patient is comfortable, verbally encourage relaxation and generally gain the patient's confidence.

It is often argued that treatment by means of EMG biofeedback is costly and very time consuming. If, on the other hand, the patient responds well to this type of treatment, surely it warrants use. Biofeedback can be combined with certain facilitatory techniques at a later stage, so that ultimately it becomes part of the re-education process and not necessarily something extra, over and above conventional therapy time.

Once the patient has learned to relax the spastic shoulder depressors and activate the prime movers, then there is no further need of the biofeedback machine. In the interim, however, it could serve a useful purpose by helping the patient gain control over his own musculature.

There still remains a number of unanswered questions and possible limitations of EMG biofeedback to be considered, particularly in respect to the neurologically involved patient. It is not yet clear when, in the course of recovery, a patient is neurophysiologically ready to use EMG biofeedback. It requires a reasonable level of conscious control and concentration and involves a number of sensory inputs, all of which may present difficulties for the early stroke patient. More has yet to be discovered, therefore, in respect to the processing of feedback information before any decision can be made in regard to optimal time application. Similarly, the level of motivation and the importance of the interaction with the therapist, in conjunction with the biofeedback machine, have yet to be determined.

CONCLUSION

EMG biofeedback has opened the way for new approaches in the treatment of the stroke patient. Although the exact anatomical and physiological pathways involved in biofeedback have yet to be determined, this modality can no doubt help to bridge a gap within the sensory feedback loop. According to Wolf (1978), a neurological patient can only re-acquire good motor control if sensory information is received and integrated correctly and proprioceptive behaviour is re-established.

From the study described (Williams, 1982), EMG biofeedback was shown to be a useful adjunct to treatment when physical therapists are attempting to decrease pain at the spastic hemiplegic shoulder. Further controlled studies are needed, however, to ascertain the optimal use of this modality, together with more emphasis on diagnosis of the cause of the shoulder pain.

REFERENCES

Amato A, Hermsmeyer C A, Kleinman K M 1973 Use of electromyographic feedback to increase inhibitory control of spastic muscles. Physical Therapy 53: 1063–1066.
Baker M, Regenos E, Wolf S L, Basmajian J V 1977 Developing strategies for biofeedback. Applications in neurologically handicapped patients. Physical Therapy 57: 402–408.
Basmajian J V, 1967 Proceedings from Northwestern University Special Therapeutic Exercise Project (NUSTEP). American Journal of Physical Therapy Medicine 46: 973–981.
Basmajian J V, Kulnulka C H, Narajan M G 1975 Biofeedback treatment of footdrop after stroke. Archives of Physical Medicine and Rehabilitation 56: 231–236.
de Bats M, de Bisschop G, Bardot A, Salmon M 1974 La subluxation inférieure de l'epaule chez l'hemiplégique. Annales de Mëdecine Physique 17: 185–213.
Bobath B 1978 Adult hemiplegia: evaluation and treatment. Heinemann, London
Brudny J, Korein J, Grynbaum B B, Friedman L W, Weinstein S, Sachs-Frankel G, Belandres P V 1976 EMG biofeedback therapy: Review of treatment of 114 patients. Archives of Physical Medicine and Rehabilitation 57: 55–61.
Brunnstrom S 1970 Movement therapy in hemiplegia. Harper and Row, New York
Bryce J M, Revised by Todd J M, Davies P M 1977 Hemiplegia II. In: J Cash (ed) Neurology for physiotherapists. Faber and Faber, London
Burnside I G, Tobias H S, Burnsill D 1979 Electromyographic feedback in remobilisation of stroke patients. In: Research in Psychology and Medicine. Academic Press, New York, pp 462–468.
Cailliet R 1978 Shoulder pain. F A Davis, Philadelphia
Cailliet R 1980 The shoulder in hemiplegia. F A Davis, Philadelphia
Chaco J, Wolf E 1971 Subluxation of the glenohumeral joint in hemiplegia. American Journal of Physical Medicine 50: 139–143.
Chino N 1981 Electrophysiological investigation on shoulder subluxation in hemiplegics. Scandinavian Journal of Rehabilitation Medicine 13: 17–21.
Codman E A 1934 The shoulder. Thomas Todd, Boston
Davis S W, Petrillo C R, Eichberg R D, Chu D S 1977 Shoulder-hand syndrome in a hemiplegic population: A 5-year retrospective study. Archives of Physical Medicine and Rehabilitation 58: 353–356.
Evans C D 1981 The practical evaluation of handicap after severe stroke. Physiotherapy 67: 199–202.

Fitzgerald-Finch, Gibson I I J 1975 Subluxation of the shoulder in hemiplegia. Age and Aging 4: 16–18.

Green A M, Green E E 1975 Biofeedback: Research and therapy. In: Jacobson O (ed) Being well is a responsibility. Turnstone Books, London

Grynbaum B B, Brudny J, Korein J, Belandres P V 1976 Sensory feedback therapy for stroke patients. Geriatrics 31: 43–47.

Harrison A, Connolly K 1971 The conscious control of fine levels of neuromuscular firing of spastic and normal subjects. Developmental Medicine and Child Neurology 13: 762–771.

Hurd W W, Pegram V, Nepomuceno C 1980 Comparison of actual and stimulated EMG biofeedback in the treatment of hemiplegic patients. American Journal of Physical Medicine 59: 73–82.

Hurrell M 1980 Electromyographic feedback in rehabilitation. Physiotherapy 66: 293–298.

Inaba M K, Piorkowski M 1972 Ultrasound in treatment of the painful shoulder in patients with hemiplegia. Physical Therapy 52: 737–741.

Jacobson E 1929 Progressive relaxation. University of Chicago Press, Chicago

Jeans M E 1979 Relief of chronic pain by brief intense, transcutaneous electrical stimulation. In: J J Bonica (ed) Advances in Pain Research and Therapy. Raven Press, New York, pp 601–606.

Jensen E M 1980 The hemiplegic shoulder. Scandinavian Journal of Rehabilitation Medicine 7: 113–119.

Johnson H E, Garton W H 1973 Muscle re-education in hemiplegia by use of an electromyographic device. Archives of Physical Medicine and Rehabilitation 54: 320–325.

Johnstone M 1978 Restoration of motor function in the stroke patient. Churchill Livingstone, Edinburgh

Kelly J L, Baker M P, Wolf S L 1979 Procedures for EMG biofeedback training in involved upper extremities of hemiplegic patients. Physical Therapy 59: 1500–1507.

Kozin E J, McCarthy D J, Sims J, Genant H 1976 The reflex sympathatetic dystrophy syndrome. The American Journal of Medicine 60: 321–331.

Marduel Y N 1980 L'epaule de l'hémiplégique. Kinésithérapie-Scientifique 182: 45–52.

Marinacci A A, Horande M 1960 Electromyogram in muscular re-education. Bulletin of the Los Angeles Neurological Society 25: 57–71.

Melzack R 1973 The puzzle of pain. Penguin Education, Harmondsworth, England

Melzack R, Casey K L 1968 Sensory, motivational and central control determinants of pain: A new conceptual model. In: D Kenshalo (ed) The skin senses. Springfield, C C Thomas, pp 423–439.

Moskowitz E 1969 Complications in the rehabilitation of hemiplegic patients. Medical Clinics of North America 53: 541–551.

Najenson T, Pikielny S S 1965 Malalignment of the gleno-humeral joint following hemiplegia. A review of 500 cases. Annals of Physical Medicine 8: 96–99.

Najenson T, Yacubovich E, Pikielny S S 1971 Rotator cuff injury in shoulder joints of hemiplegic patients. Scandinavian Journal of Rehabilitation Medicine 3: 131–137.

Nepomuceno C S, Miller J M 1974 Shoulder arthrography in hemiplegic patients. Archives of Physical Medicine and Rehabilitation 55: 49–51.

Nouwen A, Solinger J W 1979 The effectiveness of EMG biofeedback training in low back pain. Biofeedback and self-regulation 4: 103–111.

Olsson O 1953 Degenerative changes of the shoulder joint and their connective with shoulder pain. Acta Chirurgica Scandinavica 181: 34–95.

Peat M, Grahame R E 1976 An electrogoniometer for the measurement of single plane movements. Journal of Biomechanics 9: 423–424.

Swaan D, Van Wieringen P C W, Fokkema S D 1974 Auditory electromyographic feedback therapy to inhibit undesired motor activity. Archives of Physical Medicine and Rehabilitation 55: 251–254.

Todd J M 1974 Physiotherapy in the early stages of hemiplegia. Physiotherapy 60: 336–342.

Voss D 1967 Proceedings from Northwestern University Special Therapeutic Exercise Project (NUSTEP). American Journal of Physical Medicine 46: 973–981.

Walker M, Cole J 1980 Biofeedback in treatment of stroke. Australian Journal of Physiotherapy 26: 221–226.

Williams J M 1980 File search of all hemiplegic patients admitted to the Jewish Convalescent Hospital, Chomedey, Quebec, between January 1976 and March, 1979.

Williams J M 1982 Use of electromyographic biofeedback for pain reduction in the spastic hemiplegic shoulder: a pilot study. Physiotherapy Canada 34: 327–333.

Williams P L, Warwick R 1973 Gray's anatomy, 36th edn. Churchill Livingstone, London.

Wolf S L 1978 Essential considerations in the use of EMG biofeedback. Physical Therapy 58: 25–31.

Wolf S L, Baker M P, Kelly J L 1979 EMG biofeedback in stroke: effect of patient characteristics. Archives of Physical Medicine and Rehabilitation 60: 96–102.

Wolf S L, Baker M P, Kelly J L 1980 EMG biofeedback in stroke: A 1-year follow-up on the effect of patient characteristics. Archives of Physical Medicine and Rehabilitation 61: 351–355.

Zimmerman M 1979 Peripheral and central nervous mechanisms of nociception, pain and pain therapy: facts and hypothesis. In: Bonica J J (ed) Advances in Pain Research and Therapy. Raven Press, New York, pp 3–32.

The back school in an occupational setting

OCCURRENCE OF BACK TROUBLE IN WORKING LIFE

Back trouble is one of the most common causes of sick leave from work. About 10 to 15% of all the sickness absence days in Sweden are caused by back problems. It is also one of the most common causes of early retirement pension. Some 25% of all premature pensions in Sweden are due to this.

Large groups of employees have back trouble. Eight out of ten Swedes (Nachemsson, 1970; Helander, 1973) suffer from back trouble during some period of their lives. The sufferers often become more or less unable to work for long periods of time. The average sickness absence due to back trouble in Sweden is 39 days.

This entails large costs to society and large loss of production to industry. That is why it is an urgent matter to try to prevent and treat low back pain.

CAUSES OF BACK TROUBLE

The causes of back trouble are still unknown to a great extent. Body type and different deformities (e.g. scoliosis, kyphosis, leg length discrepancy) are not believed to be accountable for the high frequency of back trouble. Changes in the intervertebral discs due to age and wear, or overload of other structures in the back, have been mentioned as possible explanations.

Since the real cause of back trouble is still unknown, we concentrate for the time being on diminishing the mechanical strain on the back. It is known that certain factors in the place of work increase the occurrence of trouble and the sickness absence time (Andersson, 1979). Such factors are:
— bending and turning of the back
— static working positions
— sudden high physical workloads

— heavy physical work (lifting)
— vibrations.

Many sufferers are also of the opinion that the causes of the trouble are to be found in the work environment. In a recent Danish study (Biering-Söerensen, 1983), slightly more than half of the sufferers said that the trouble was connected to their jobs. In a corresponding Swedish study in heavy industry (Heibel, 1978), every third person reported that they experienced stress on the back in their jobs.

This knowledge has had the result that we in Sweden, during the last years, have invested many resources in trying to prevent back trouble. Through ergonomic improvements of the work place and through teaching preventive back care we hope to be able to diminish the mechanical strain on the back in working life and at the same time the frequency of trouble. The Swedish Occupational Health Service has a key role in this work.

SWEDISH OCCUPATIONAL HEALTH SERVICE

Originally, the Occupational Health Service in Sweden concentrated on preventing accidents and giving 'medical care' to the employees. At the beginning of the 50s, the goals of the Occupational Health Service were changed by an increased interest in preventive work. They started by improving working conditions for the employees such as eliminating unnecessary loads on muscles and joints. In that way ergonomics became an important field of activities for the Occupational Health Service.

The Swedish Occupational Health Service is based on voluntary contracts between the parties of the labour market. The aim of the activities are as follows:
— protect employees from health hazards on the job (accidents and occupational diseases)
— work toward optimal job adaptation and optimal working conditions from the view of human needs and capacities (ergonomics)
— contribute toward the restoration of health and working capacity as soon as possible following accidents and disease (rehabilitation)
— integrate health and production considerations.

The Occupational Health Service thus contains both technical and medical prevention, and treatment and rehabilitation. Organizationally, the Occupational Health Service usually consists of a technical sector with industrial safety engineers and a medical sector with company physicians, nurses and physical therapists. More and more importance is attached to preventive work. The Occupational Health Service has a very important consultative function in connection with purchasing of machinery and other types of working equipment and with production planning. Another important part of preventive activities is teaching about work environment problems for different categories of employees.

THE ROLE OF THE PHYSICAL THERAPIST IN THE OCCUPATIONAL HEALTH SERVICE AND IN PREVENTIVE WORK

Only recently has the physical therapist been included in the Occupational Health Service. The first physical therapist to work in the Occupational Health Service in the 1950s and 60s was mainly concerned with rehabilitation. But during the 70s she has gradually become more engaged in preventive work. Because of her knowledge of anatomy and physiology the physical therapist is regarded as well qualified to analyze the connection between pain and work load, and to make ergonomic judgments of the place of work. Today, about 350 physical therapists work within Swedish industry and another 250 in the Occupational Health Service within the government.

In addition to their physical therapy basic training these physical therapists usually have additional training in Occupational Health Service practices and in ergonomics. The training includes 5 intensive weeks, a literature review and a special written assignment in ergonomics.

In a recent investigation concerning occupational health, this specialized education is proposed to be lengthened to 6 months.

The Swedish physical therapists working in the Occupational Health Service are organized in a society which arranges conferences and provides further training in ergonomics, biomechanics, physiology of exercise, pedagogics and psychology. Organizationally, the physical therapist usually belongs to the medical section of the Occupational Health Service, but she can also be independently responsible for an ergonomic section. Her duties at work are prevention as well as rehabilitation and treatment. The preventive work consists mainly of teaching ergonomics and working techniques to the employees conducting ergonomic surveys and evaluations of work places and of analyzing connections between work and pain and proposing preventive measures. In the ergonomic work she collaborates closely with the industrial safety engineers.

Physical therapy treatment and rehabilitation within the Occupational Health Service consists of taking care of employees with job-related diseases and pain, i.e. trouble caused by or aggravated by their job. This means that the main part of treatment involves taking care of employees suffering from troubles in the low back, neck and shoulders. Many patients also have stress-related trouble, such as muscle tension and headaches caused by tension.

Therefore, work with back schools, neck schools and relaxation groups are an important part of the physical therapist's job in an occupational setting.

BACK SCHOOL—HISTORY

In the beginning of the 1970s a physical therapist named Marianne Zachrisson-Forsell had the idea to help patients with back trouble by teaching them in groups. In groups she gave basic instruction on how to treat backs in order to prevent trouble. The back school proved to be a more effective substitute for other methods of treatment that had little if any effect on recovery since most patients recover spontaneously. The back school is based on the idea that increased load gives increased trouble.

Marianne Zachrisson-Forsell set the following aims for the back school:
— to increase the individual's ability to take care of his back
— to prevent back trouble
— to teach the individual to make the best out of his situation in spite of his back trouble.

Marianne Zachrisson-Forsell worked out an audiovisual program consisting of four lessons. The use of this film-strip has been widespread in Sweden and abroad.

The value of the back school was confirmed by Marianne Bergqvist Ullman (1977) who did a comparative study at the Volvo car factory among employees with acute or sub-acute back pain. She showed that those who had participated in the back school had shorter periods of pain and lower sickness absence compared to patients who had received only conventional physical therapy or only short-wave diathermy treatment.

During the last few years, different forms of back schools have been established in Sweden in hospitals as well as in the Occupational Health Service. Marianne Zachrisson-Forsell's original back

school is still used in many places of work but many physical therapists have also developed modified programs to meet the needs of
their own patients' working situations. There are back schools especially adapted to different branches of industry, ranging from
building to forestry. The original back school was aimed at secondary prevention, i.e. to help those who had chronic or acute back
trouble. In the last few years the back school, within the Occupational Health Service, has also begun primary prevention and focuses on groups of employees who have no established back
trouble.

Both the primary and secondary schools reach large groups of
employees. Ergonomic advising is an important feature of the teaching; the students probably pass on some of this knowledge to their
companions. Thus, the back school becomes even more important
in adapting the specific job, and it becomes normative to the ergonomic design of other places of work.

OCCUPATIONAL HEALTH SERVICE AND
PRESERVATION OF HEALTH AT SAAB-SCANIA

Saab-Scania is one of the major industries in Sweden. The company
manufactures civil and military aircraft. The company has extensive
health services which provide over 6500 employees with medical
care, care for preservation of health, rehabilitation therapy and
technical safety service. There are two physical therapists employed
and I am one of them.

In our company it has been a tradition to make large investments
in preservation of the employees' health and rehabilitation. In 1975,
when I was hired as the first physical therapist of the company, a
physical training centre with a rehabilitation facility and a health
preservation program had already been established. The facilities
were conveniently housed under the same roof (Fig. 9.1).

In the physical training centre, a close collaboration has developed between the company physical therapists and the personnel
in charge of the care for preservation of health. We offer activities
for elite athletes, 'fitness freaks' and ordinary joggers, as well as
rehabilitation patients.

The goal of integrating patients with 'healthy' people is to create
an environment emphasizing fitness as opposed to illness. Employees can receive help with weight-loss, smoking cessation and physical training, and at the same time they are encouraged to take

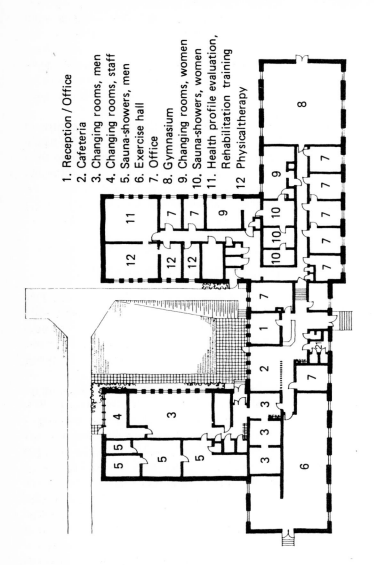

1. Reception / Office
2. Cafeteria
3. Changing rooms, men
4. Changing rooms, staff
5. Sauna-showers, men
6. Exercise hall
7. Office
8. Gymnasium
9. Changing rooms, women
10. Sauna-showers, women
11. Health profile evaluation,
    Rehabilitation training
12. Physicaltherapy

Fig. 9.1 Saab Scania Physical Training Centre

greater responsiblity for their own health. The physical therapy activities are based on the following guiding principles:

— Take care of patients as early as possible. No long waiting lists.
— Treat with a comprehensive approach. An evaluation of the total health condition and working situation is a natural part of the procedure.
— Consult without an appointment. The employees can phone or come in for consultation any time during office hours.
— Devote no more than 50% of working hours to medical treatment. The emphasis is on prevention.
— Make the patients responsible for their training at an early stage. They are given individually tailored training programs to follow during their training in our exercise hall.
— Regularly schedule back school, neck school and relaxation groups.
— As soon as possible, place patients under the care of the physical training staff for a conditioning test and further help with their training.

BACK-REHABILITATION PROGRAM AT SAAB-SCANIA

Back trouble is a relatively common complaint among our employees. Recently, a survey of 10% of our employees about leisure time activities and the working environment showed that 35% of these had had back trouble during the last 3 months, 28% had had trouble on rare occasions and 7% suffered often or very often. In an inquiry on absenteeism carried out in 1978, we found that about 4% of the employees had missed more than 7 days that year due to back problems. Our results are comparable to the figures of a study at Volvo among men aged 40 to 47 (Svensson-Andersson 1982) which indicated that 30% had back trouble at the time of the investigation, and that about 4% had chronic or severe trouble. These studies show that there is a large group of employees who could benefit from the back school's teachings.

For these reasons we have formed a special rehabilitation program in our company (Fig. 9.2). The program is based on the fact that the working environment is directly connected to the patient's back problem and should be evaluated if he is receiving treatment. The aim of the physical therapist, then, is to determine if there is a connection between the patient's complaints and some ergonomic factor at the work place.

Our program contains different steps so that the treatment can

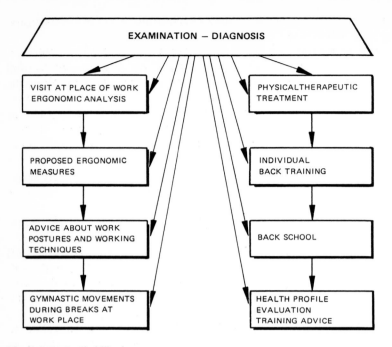

Fig. 9.2 Back-rehabilitation program

include one or several measures. On the patient's first visit we examine him and take his history including questions concerning his working environment and leisure time activities. On the basis of this information we decide if our patient needs any form of individual physical therapy treatment, a training program or if he can go directly to the back school. We also decide if we should visit the patient's work place.

For example, a patient with lumbago ischias is first treated with traction and then progresses to the back school. Another patient who suffers from low back strain or a patient with subacute lumbago may go directly to the back school. Other patients start with a physical training program; one such patient with chronic lumbago has been given numerous treatments with little or no effect. For these kinds of patients we form individually adapted training programs. The program usually consists of a warm-up on a bicycle ergometer and different kinds of exercises in order to improve strength and physical fitness. For these programs we use dumbells and other kinds of modern training apparatus. The patient is then allowed to train for 1 hour per day during paid working hours, 2 to 3 times a week for 5 to 6 weeks. These patients can also continue in the back school.

After this training our patients are encouraged to continue to train during their leisure time in our physical training centre. We give them advice and instructions on how to carry on with different forms of training. Some continue individual training in our gymnasium or on our 1 km track. Others continue to train in a group and can participate in some of the gymnastics groups we have during lunch hours or in the training group we have for former back school patients one evening a week.

SAAB-SCANIA'S BACK SCHOOL

Saab-Scania's back school was formed in 1977. Based on Marianne Zachrisson-Forsell's original back school, it was modified with regard to the specific environmental problems of our company and the resources available at the Training Centre. Today, our back school is based on the use of the variety of training methods available in the centre, since the back school staff and the fitness centre staff are in close collaboration.

The students come to the back school on the recommendation of the company doctor, their foreman or safety representative. The back school is run during paid working hours. The people participating are usually not sick listed. About 80 employees participate in the back school every year. The aim of the back school is to teach the patients to alleviate current pain and to prevent new pain. Its aim is to give the participants:

— knowledge of the anatomy and function of the back
— increased consciousness of their backs and an understanding of the causes of strain on their backs
— knowledge of, and experience in, proper work-related techniques and postures
— an understanding of how their places of work and home environments can be improved to minimize problem-causing situations
— lessons on suitable gymnastic movements for the back and insight into the importance of regular exercise.

Our back school consists of 6 lessons (Fig. 9.3). The students are taught in groups of 6 to 8 persons and the teaching is based on a mixture of theory, practical exercises and group discussions. Each lesson is 60 minutes.

The first three lessons begin with 10–15 minutes of theory during

Lesson 1	The anatomy and function of the back. Different causes of back trouble. Suitable resting postures.
Lesson 2	Load on the back by standing and sedentary work postures. Function of the muscles. Gymnastic movements for the back.
Lesson 3	Principles for lifts. Practical training of lifts and working techniques. Gymnastics.
Lesson 4	Ergonomics of the place of work. Check-list for evaluation of the place of work. Gymnastics for the back.
Lesson 5	Physical training by back pain. Training program for the back. Stretching exercises.
Lesson 6	Revision and summary. Gymnastics, jogging or walk.
	Health profile evaluation

Fig. 9.3 Back school program

which Marianne Zachrisson-Forsell's filmstrip is shown. A discussion with the participants about the contents follows.

Every lesson concludes with some exercises for the back.

Lesson 1

The film-strip on the anatomy and function of the back is shown to the students. Possible causes of the individual's trouble are then illuminated. The spinal column and parts of the skeleton with vertebrae and intervertebral discs are shown. The physical therapist and the students discuss the problems of the back with regard to causes, prognosis and different methods of treatment available. At the end of the lesson the students try different rest and load-relieving positions for the back.

Lesson 2

This lesson begins with the film-strip showing how the load on the back varies with different sedentary and standing working postures.

The function of the muscles of the back are illustrated. The physical therapist then shows pictures of different groups of muscles supporting the back and she points out the importance of exercising them. She tries to explain the connection between pain, anxiety and muscular tension to the students and they are given the opportunity to discuss their own problems.

Finally, the physical therapist demonstrates exercises for the abdominal muscles and other supporting musculature which can be practised at home. The lesson is terminated by 10 minutes of gymnastics set to music.

Lesson 3

The third part of the film-strip is shown. This lesson deals with the sedentary and standing working position. The students are taught how to treat their backs for acute back trouble and the proper way to get into and out of bed. After the theoretical instruction the students practise transfer of weight, and they apply these movements to daily situations.

We discuss and practise lifting techniques and the lifting problems that the individuals themselves have in their daily lives.

The students are given instructions for developing their leg muscles, and are taught additional movements that they can practise at home. Again gymnastics to music completes the lesson.

Lesson 4

During this lesson we show no pictures but devote our time to discussing the ergonomic problems that the individuals may have in their working places. We show different chairs for office and workship use and the students learn to adjust them to best suit themselves.

We also emphasize the importance of working in the best posture, and use a table of variable height to demonstrate. The students have the opportunity to adjust the table to a suitable working level for themselves, both standing and sitting. We also discuss different aids for improving working positions, e.g. foot stools, elbow-rests, copy holders and so on. The students are given a check-list (Fig. 9.4) to take to their own working places, so they can evaluate them from an ergonomic point of view and suggest possible improvements.

CHECK-LIST

1. Do you think your back pain has any connection with your present work?

Yes, absolutely ☐
Yes, maybe ☐
Probably not ☐
No, absolutely not ☐

2. If not, is there any other probable reason for your trouble, e.g. your spare time activities?

. . . .

3 If yes, do you think your trouble is due to:

	Yes	No
Heavy working movements, e.g. lifts	☐	☐
Prolonged bent or turned work posture	☐	☐
One-sided sedentary or standing work posture	☐	☐

4. Evaluate your place of work with regard to following factors:

	Very good	Acceptable	Not acceptable
Working height	☐	☐	☐
Placing of working materials	☐	☐	☐
Control and instruments placing	☐	☐	☐
Working chair	☐	☐	☐
Room for legs	☐	☐	☐
Lighting	☐	☐	☐
Floor base	☐	☐	☐

5. Is there lifting work at your work place? ☐ Yes ☐ No

If yes, how often do you lift? . . . .

How heavy lifts? . . . .

6. Would you like the physicaltherapist come and look at your work place?

. . . .

Fig. 9.4 Back school check-list

Like the other lessons, this lesson is terminated by a gymnastics program for about 15 minutes.

Lesson 5

In the fifth lesson we concentrate on physical training, and begin with a discussion on exercises and types of training that can be done

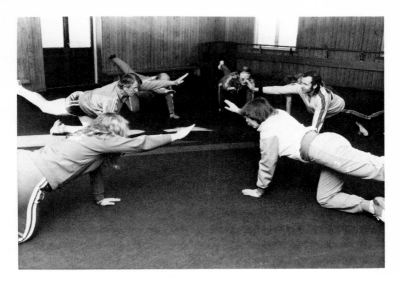

Plate 9.1 The physical therapist instructs her back school students in gymnastic movements

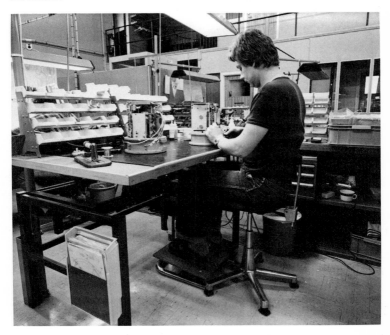

Plate 9.2 As a result of attending the back school this employee's workplace has been ergonomically improved

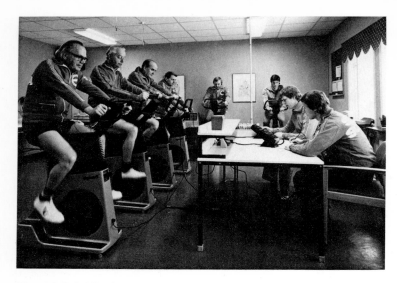

Plate 9.3 Rehabilitation patients at Saab Scania exercise on ergocycle during paid working hours

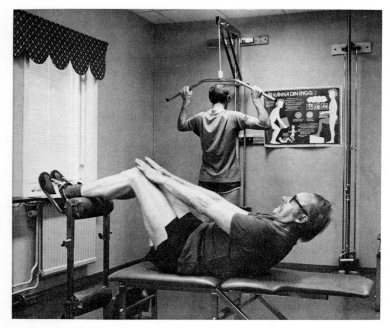

Plate 9.4 Back school students train their back and abdominal muscles in the exercise hall.

to avoid back and neck trouble. This lesson is also attended by a representative of the fitness staff. We walk over to the exercise hall of the physical training centre where we and the fitness instructor demonstrate and the students are given the chance to try a program especially adapted for back training. Finally, they are taught some stretching exercises for the hamstrings, calves and back muscles.

Lesson 6

The last lesson gives a revision of the back school training program. We show a selection of slides about the back and scenes from environments similar to those in which our students work. We put questions to them and discuss individual problems.

The check-lists that our students have completed are handed in and discussed, and the individuals are given advice on possible improvements. The physical therapist will make a follow-up visit to the workplace if the individual wishes. Finally, the students receive a written summary with illustrations on all they have learned. It contains, for example, advice about resting postures, working techniques and working postures, plus a program for training the back, to be used at home.

HEALTH PROFILE EVALUATION

After attending the back school, all the students are summoned to the physical training centres for health screening. The health profile check-up has been developed by Sture Malmgren at Saab-Scania and is the basis of our health promotion program. The screening consists of a questionnaire regarding the student's lifestyle which can be transformed into a graphical description (Fig. 9.5), and is called a health profile.

Blood pressure and skeletal weight are measured in accordance with von Döbeln's method (von Döbeln, 1960) and a submaximal exercise test is administered on an ergocycle. The questionnaire and test results become the basis for the evaluation of physical working capacity, body composition and lifestyle.

In a final discussion, the test leader helps the participant interpret the physiological values measured in the screening process. A contract is drawn up regarding desired changes in training, smoking, or eating. It is the participant's responsibility to decide specifically what, when and how he wants to change his poor habits.

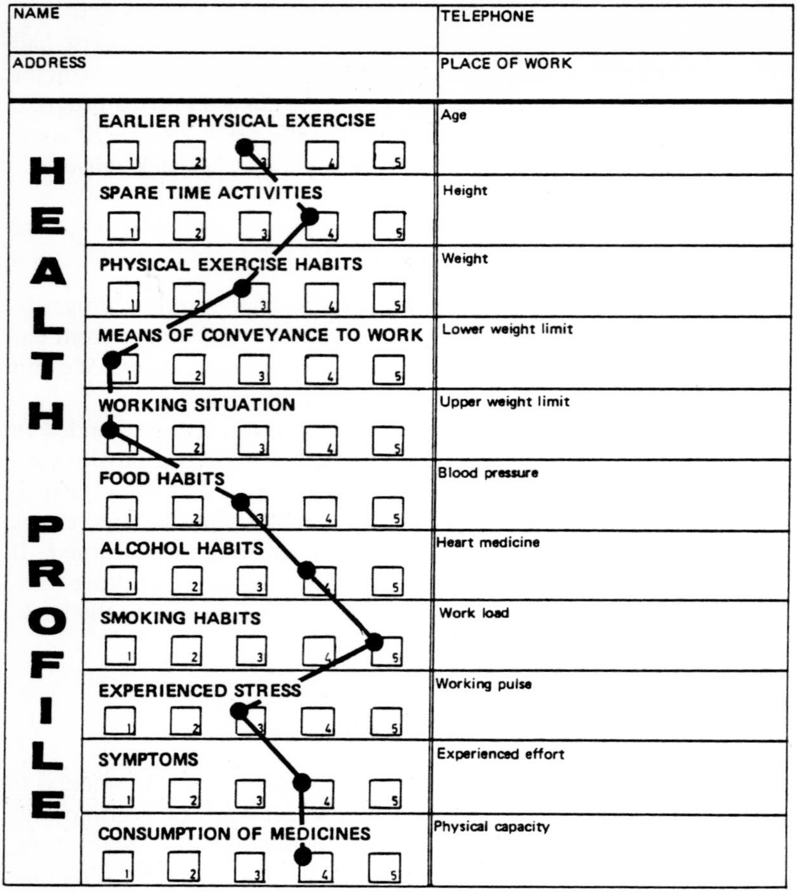

NAME		TELEPHONE
ADDRESS		PLACE OF WORK

		Age
H	EARLIER PHYSICAL EXERCISE □1 □2 ■3 □4 □5	Age
E	SPARE TIME ACTIVITIES □1 □2 □3 ■4 □5	Height
A	PHYSICAL EXERCISE HABITS □1 ■2 □3 □4 □5	Weight
L	MEANS OF CONVEYANCE TO WORK ■1 □2 □3 □4 □5	Lower weight limit
T		
H	WORKING SITUATION ■1 □2 □3 □4 □5	Upper weight limit
P	FOOD HABITS □1 □2 ■3 □4 □5	Blood pressure
R	ALCOHOL HABITS □1 □2 □3 ■4 □5	Heart medicine
O	SMOKING HABITS □1 □2 □3 □4 ■5	Work load
F	EXPERIENCED STRESS □1 □2 ■3 □4 □5	Working pulse
I		
L	SYMPTOMS □1 □2 □3 ■4 □5	Experienced effort
E	CONSUMPTION OF MEDICINES □1 □2 □3 ■4 □5	Physical capacity

Fig. 9.5 Health profile evaluation

The health profile has several important objectives (Fig. 9.6), but the three major points are:
— to motivate the individual to improve his lifestyle with regard to health experience and physical data
— to survey and follow up the high risk groups: smokers and those with low physical activity levels and a high percentage of body fat
— to catch individuals in need of a closer examination for special training later on.

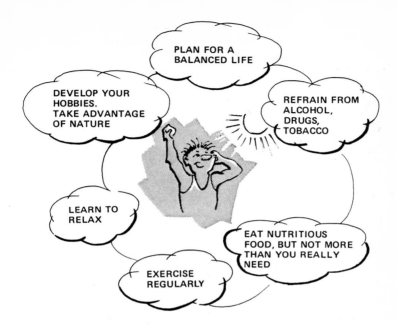

Fig. 9.6 Pay attention to your health profile

QUESTIONNAIRE AND FIELD INVESTIGATION CONCERNING THE BACK SCHOOL

We have studied the back school at Saab-Scania (Myrnerts, 1982), in order to describe how the participants reacted to the different components of the school and to find out if the presentations led to a decrease in back problems. We also wanted to find out if the back school resulted in any changes in working techniques and exercise habits. The first investigation was done in 1980 among 180 participants of the back school during 1978 to 1979. This study led to the following changes in the back school:

— The theoretical element was reduced in favour of the practical training in movement and working techniques.
— A health profile evaluation became routine after the back school.
— A check-list was formed to simplify students' evaluations of their workplaces and to stimulate their interest in changing their own work environment.

Another field investigation was conducted in 1981 comprising 100 participants in the back school. Later in the same year this study was supplemented with interviews on health and exercise for 23 of the original 100 participants. With this additional information we could evaluate some of the motives for behavioral changes.

THE BACK-SCHOOL GROUP

The average age of the participants was 45 years. 83% were men and 17% were women. 65% were white-collar workers and the rest were blue-collar workers. These figures correspond closely to the distribution of employees within our company. In our interview group we randomly chose proportional numbers from each category to discover any differences between white and blue collar workers.

CONTENTS OF THE BACK SCHOOL

In our field investigations, the students were asked to evaluate the different parts of the back school. We found that the participants felt that all the information was important, but the most beneficial was the information given about working posture. They reported that they often used better lifting and working techniques after attending the back school.

In other words, the group placed more importance on the basic discussion about the strains on the back and the practical training than on the theoretical parts of the lessons. One member said: 'I'm one of those who never want much theory; I want to do more practical things. I want to have *some* basic theory to understand what I am doing, though.'

Many studies have shown that theoretical knowledge disappears quickly and according to modern pedagogic principles, concentration should be on instructing basic principles instead of on little sections of knowledge. Too many facts are confusing, and should therefore be limited. Modern educational theories also stress that the education should be oriented to individual problems and experiences, and pupils should be activated as much as possible. The more active the pupil, the better his learning and retention.

In organising the back school, we have tried to reduce the theoretical element in favour of practical training and discussion of individual problems.

EXPERIENCED IMPROVEMENT OF BACK PAIN

One of the purposes of the back school is to alleviate back pain. 73% of our students (Fig. 9.7) felt that the trouble had lessened

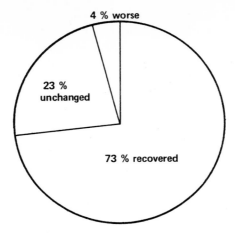

Fig. 9.7 Back pain after the Saab Scania back school

after attending the back school. 23% said there had been no change and 4% felt that the pains had increased. Similar results have been found by others. 'The Canadian Back Education units' (Hall, 1980) reported that 77% of the participants experienced improvements. The majority of our participants were of the opinion that the improvement was a result of their increased awareness of their backs, of improving their lifting and working techniques and of continuing rehabilitation exercises.

The frequency of recurrence among back patients is high. During our interviews it appeared that many people occasionally experience increased pain. The Volvo study shows that 60% had recurrences within a year, but those who had participated in Volvo's back school had less pain and shorter periods of pain than others. During interviews, 1 to 1¼ years after our back school, we asked our students if they perceived their back problems as a hindrance to daily activity. 70% felt their pain was not an obstacle to daily activity. For them it could be that an increase in back trouble functions as an alarm-clock. They say that when they feel the pain appearing, they become more conscious of their posture.

About one-third also perform the gymnastic movements they learned in the back school. One of the most important motivational factors, according to Madsen (1975) and Castle & Kobbs (1966), is the desire to avoid pain. One individual expressed it like this: 'I am motivated to exercise when I have pain, it's so easy to postpone the exercise when I don't feel my back.'

The level of anxiety also effects the pain perceived, and the reduction of anxiety is a very important part of our teaching. Anxiety can stem from uncertainty about the problem. 25% of the pupils we interviewed said that they felt anxiety. All except one said that this anxiety lessened considerably after the back school. This is well illustrated by the following quotations: 'I am less worried now because I learned how I could help myself get better,' 'Earlier I was worried about how I would manage my leisure activities, my garden and things like that.'

We think, therefore, that it is very important to discuss the course of the disease and its prognosis and also explain to the group the connection between anxiety, pain and muscular tension.

Finally, the students are given the opportunity to discuss their own experiences of pain.

CHANGED WORKING TECHNIQUES

A large part of our teaching in the back school is aimed at teaching the participants better lifting and working techniques. It is very difficult to study the changes in people's working techniques in an objective way, since conditions previous to attendance must be

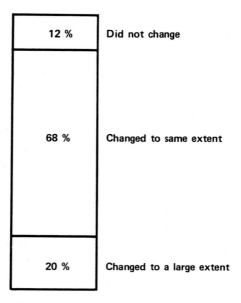

Fig. 9.8 Changes of working techniques

examined. Therefore, there is a great risk that our results reflect more the attitudes of the individuals than their real changes of behaviour.

In our inquiry, 20% claimed that they had improved their working techniques (Fig. 9.8) considerably, 68% to some extent and 12% not at all. Apparently, the practical training has had some effect on this behaviour. This can also be shown by the following quotations from our interviews: 'To think before lifting is a must now.' 'I got a living demonstration of how to move in different situations.' 'I am much more aware of how I am sitting now.'

We have found that the knowledge about working techniques is often spread at the places of work. Foremen, instructors and others often pass on their knowledge of 'how to sit, lift, stand' to their working companions. The physical therapists also hold classes to teach the supervisors proper techniques for their workers.

CHANGES IN THE WORK ENVIROMENT

Our study showed that 40% of our students saw a connection between their back trouble and their work. Slightly more than 80% of them were of the opinion that work posture was the cause. It is particularly interesting to note that almost half of them had sedentary jobs. Only a small number had jobs which were physically demanding. The often one-sided working postures and work movements that occur doing sedentary work seem to put considerable strain on the back.

In our first inquiry we asked the participants if there had been any ergonomic changes made at their work places after the back school. 29% answered yes to this question. This often meant getting a better chair or changing the adjustment of the chair they had. In a very few cases, a change to the working height of a machine or a table had been made. Slightly more than half of the students had taken the initiative to make these changes themselves. The others had received help from the physical therapist.

In view of the fact that so many people believed in a connection between their environment and their back trouble, we saw a need for more ergonomic improvements. In an attempt to increase the interest in this among our students, we introduced a check-list (Fig. 9.4). They receive the check-list during the fourth lesson that deals with technical design of the work place. The results of the work place evaluations are then discussed during the last lesson.

In 1981 we studied the effect of introducing the check-list. We found that the use of the check-list had not entailed any increase in the number of changes in the work environment. The physical therapist had still initiated almost half of the changes made.

During our interviews we tried to discover the reasons for this. We asked our students if they thought that they had an influence on their work environment. We found that there was a difference between white collar workers and blue collar workers. The white collar workers stated that they usually had the opportunity to improve their working environment. For example, after learning about the importance of having a good chair, most had no difficulty in getting a new one. On the other hand, the blue collar workers who experienced trouble with their working environments often had difficulty in bringing about changes. The design of the machinery, lack of funds and lack of understanding were obstacles frequently mentioned. There were also obstacles of a psychological nature. Some expressed it like this: 'I'm afraid of being a nagger and a complainer.' 'If I have a new chair, everybody else must have one too.' The conclusion we have drawn from this is that it is difficult for the individual employee, particularly for the blue collar worker, to initiate changes in his work environment. If necessary changes are to be made, the physical therapist must visit the work place. This opportunity to follow-up and analyze the working situation is unique for the occupational health physical therapist, and we see it as one of her most valuable functions. This personal interest combined with ergonomic knowledge will stimulate concern and understanding about work place problems among foremen and others.

It may be necessary to carry out many different types of changes in a place of work in order to make it a more comfortable, friendlier place for the back. Desired changes may include: raising a machine, changing the location of a control lever, improving the handling of materials, introducing elbow rests, angling a work-board or altering the lighting. These changes require money and, of course, assistance from foremen and production engineers. This is part of the reason why it is so important for the physical therapist in an occupational setting to be in close collaboration with these groups.

We have kept our check-list, but its primary use is as a basis for discussion between the physical therapist, the worker and the foreman. It also gives us a reason for follow-up.

CHANGED EXERCISE HABITS

Prolonged back pain often leads to reduced physical activity with the resulting deterioration of physical condition, muscular endurance and strength. This is one of the reasons why we have included exercise as an important element in our back school. We want students to become more active and give them a better physical tolerance.

As part of our follow-up evaluation we sent out a questionnaire which defined physical training as 'physical activity in training clothes with the purpose of improving one's physical or general condition'. In our results, we found that about 25% had increased their exercise level. In our interviews, we found that as many as half of the students said they had improved their exercise habits. The ones who had increased their physical training were mainly those who had been sporadically active before the back school or who had done some training once or twice weekly. Only a few people who had been inactive had started training regularly. Most said that the main reasons for this change were that they had been motivated by the back school and that they were given a proper training format.

Those who had experienced an alleviation of back pain and a general sense of well-being in connection with their training, were more motivated than others to continue. Some comments were: 'I felt that I could strengthen and cure my back by exercising; if it is this easy that I can train for 10 minutes a day and then get rid of my back pain, then I think it is really worthwhile trying.' 'I feel more content with myself when I do some training.'

8% of our participants, however, had reduced their training. Reasons included increased back trouble, shortage of time and lack of interest.

Those who did not exercise at all gave similar reasons. They said for example: 'I'm too tired after work.' 'I never get around to it.' 'I don't think physical training will help me.'

Most of the students continue the exercises they learned in the back school, and half do them regularly. 25% jog, and many cycle or walk. Others keep fit by exercising in groups, body-building or swimming.

Our results show that our investment in different forms of physical activity has given our students a stimulus and motivated them to start and continue training.

Another important factor in this context is our location. While in the back school, individuals have the chance to meet some of the physical training centre's fitness staff and they become familiar with the premises and the facilities available. If they feel at home in the environment it is much easier for them to continue training either in groups or individually.

SOME PEDAGOGIC ASPECTS

One of the aims of the back school is to change certain attitudes and behaviors that are common among those with back problems. In order to make these changes we use modern pedagogic principles.

Some of these positive pedagogic components in our back school are:

— Groups are limited to 6 to 8 persons. This facilitates communication within the group and creates a supportive atmosphere.
— Presentations are easy to understand. The terminology can easily be understood by the average person.
— The members are encouraged to discuss their own problems and often give practical hints and advice to one another.
— The theoretical component is limited and deals mainly with the basic principles of back treatment.
— The teaching emphasizes the importance of exercise, and all are expected to participate actively.
— The last lesson includes a summary and a question-and-answer session where the students try to answer each other's questions.

In order to attain maximum retention in both practice and theory, it is important that the school is supplemented by additional meetings. Most of the people who answered our inquiries said that they wanted a follow-up. We have now begun follow-ups and we summon our students for a lesson about 6 months to one year after completion of the the back school. In connection with this follow-up they are summoned for a new health profile evaluation.

SUMMARY

Back trouble is one of the major causes of absenteeism in industry. Many of these problems are caused or aggravated by working postures. In the last decade the Swedish physical therapists working within the Occupational Health Service have had a key role in the task of preventing back problems and in rehabilitation when they do occur. Through work with back schools and ergonomic training the physical therapist can improve the employees' working techniques and environment, and in these ways lessen the strain on the back.

Saab-Scania is one of the largest companies in Sweden and a special back rehabilitation program has been created for the employees. The program consists of physical therapy and a back school. The back school consists of 6 lessons and is held at Saab-Scania's physical training centre. Here the physical therapists work in close collaboration with physical training instructors.

The back school is based on modern pedagogic principles which emphasize practical and theoretical applications. It also points out the importance of physical exercise, good working techniques and an ergonomically designed working environment. When a person enters the the back school his physical fitness and general well-being are evaluated with a health profile designed by members of our physical training staff. This evaluation includes an ergocycle test and a lifestyle questionnaire. We hope that a concrete evaluation will stimulate our patients to improve their condition and change poor habits.

Our follow-up investigations have shown that 73% of our pupils experienced improvement in their back problems after attending the back school. We have also shown that many people exercise more regularly and have become more active, but motivation is difficult for those who have not previously been involved in exercise.

Ergonomic advice concerning the pupils' working techniques and work place, plays an important role in the back school. In a follow-up survey, most of our patients (68%) said that they had changed their working techniques. We also found that 40% believe that there is a connection between their back trouble and their work. As a rule, they find it hard to change their working environments. We teach our students basic ergonomic principles and to make a simple investigation of their own work place. Our investigations have shown that this is not enough to decrease all of the problems as much as possible, and some improvements in the working environment are necessary. The physical therapist must follow-up her patients at their work places, analyze their working environment, and suggest necessary ergonomic improvements.

REFERENCES

Andersson G 1979 Low back pain in industry: Epidemiological aspects. Scandinavian Journal of Rehabilitation Medicine 11: 163–168
Bergquist-Ullman M, Larsson U 1977 Acute low back pain in industry. Acta Orthopaedica Scandinavica. Supplement 170
Biering-Sörensen 1983 A prospective study of low back pain in a general population. Scandinavian Journal of Rehabilitation Medicine 15: 71–96

von Döbel W 1960 Mätmetoder och nomenklatur. Läkertidningen nr. 36
  Stockholm
Hall H 1980 The Canadian back education units. Physiotherapy 66: 115–117
Heibel C A 1978 Occurrence of personal handicaps in an industrial population,
  survey and appraisal. Scandinavian Journal of Rehabilitation Medicine.
  Supplement 6
Helander E 1973 Back disability and work inability. Social medicinsk Tidskrift
  50:378 (in Swedish)
Kasl S V 1966 Health behavior, illness behavior and sick roll behavior. Archives
  on Environmental Health 12
Madsen K 1975 Motivation-drivkraften bakom våra handling-Stockholm
Malmgren S, Andersson G 1976 På jakt efter hälsoprofilen. Socialmed inst.
  Universitet i Linköping
Marton-Dahlgren 1974 Inlrning och omvärldsuppfattning AWE/Gebers Stockholm
Myrnerts G 1982 The Saab Scania Back School-an evaluation. Proceedings from
  the IX International Congress for Physical Therapy, Stockholm, Sweden p. 553
Myrnerts G, Thunberg M Saab Scanias Ryggskola-en interv-juundersökning
  rörande motiv och hinder för beteende förändringar. Pedagog inst. Universitet i
  Linköping
Nachemsson A 1970 New aspects on low back pain. Forskning och praktik 2:3
  (in Swedish)
Nachemsson A Low back pain-its etiology and treatment. Clinical Medicine 78:18
Svensson H, Andersson G 1982 Low back pain in 40–47 year old men
  Frequency of occurrence and impact on medical services. Scandinavian Journal
  of Rehabilitation Medicine 14: 47–53
Zachrisson-Forsell M 1980 The Swedish back school. Physiotherapy 66: 112–114
Zachrisson-Forsell M 1981 The back school. Spine 6: 104–106
Åstrand, P-O & Rodahl, K 1977 Textbook of work physiology 2nd edn McGraw-
  Hill, New York, pp 343–352

The pain clinic approach

It is one o'clock on a January day and Mr Jones has just arrived for his
appointment with Dr Gray, his family physician. The receptionist observes Mr
Jones for a few minutes, then pulls his file from the cabinet. It is not difficult to
find because it is the thickest one on file. He has been here many times, always
with the same complaint of pain in his right hip.

As the nurse watches him, she observes that he is sitting in the waiting room in
a relatively comfortable-looking position as he pages through a magazine. He
looks up and smiles when he notices she is looking at him. 'Hmmm', she thinks
to herself, 'this guy can't be in as much pain as he always says he is.'

An hour later Dr Gray approaches examining room No. 3, and reaches for the
patient's chart carefully placed on the shelf to the left of the door. Even before he
reads the name on the file, he knows by its thickness to whom it belongs. 'Mr
Jones is back?' he winces. 'What more can I do for him!!!'

'Hi, Mr Jones. It's good to see you again. What brings you in today?' (As if I
did not know.)

'It's nothing new. This pain in my hip is really killing me. Isn't there
something else you can do?'

'Let's see. In the last three or four years . . .'

'Five and a half years,' interrupts Mr. Jones.

'Hmmm, has it been that long? Let's see. The neurologist did an EMG and a
nerve conduction velocity study. But everything was normal' the doctor said.

'Was that the thing with needles?' asked Mr. Jones.

The doctor nods affirmatively.

'I remember! I hurt extra for two weeks after that!'

'X-rays, all normal. Cat-scan, normal. Physical therapy didn't seem to help',
said the doctor, reading from the chart.

'Oh, those massages really felt good for a while.'

'The transcutaneous electrical nerve stimulator helped you, but your skin broke
out in a rash and your wife said it made you more irritable, so we had to stop
that. The myelogram showed some disk problems; surgery, however, did not
relieve your pain. The cortisone injection did not help. I have tried you on all the
medications that I know of which should help. But you say, nothing helps' the
doctor said.

'Some of them made me so drowsy, I just couldn't stay awake. The one you
have me on now seems to make me hurt worse.'

'Before you came to me, you saw a chiropractor, a rolfer, and an acupuncturist,
is that right?'

'Yes,' Mr Jones replied.

'But they didn't help you either?' asked the doctor.

'No,' Mr Jones said, with the color draining out of his cheeks. Suddenly he
looked several decades older than his 33 years.

'We've tried everything I know of to try. You should have been better a long time ago. How about my sending you to the pain clinic? Maybe they can do something for you.'

'What is that?'

'It's a clinic that treats patients with pain like yours.'

This same scenario repeats itself about a hundred times each month in doctor's offices and clinics all over the country. A physician, unable to successfully treat the chronic pain patient with conventional methods, often grasps at the opportunity to send the patient to someone else. His busy medical practice will not miss this patient; in fact, he finds it much more rewarding to treat patients who can be helped by conventional medical methods.

The referring physician really does not know what the pain clinic is or what it does that helps the chronic pain patient, but he is willing to give it a try. The patient does not really know what it is either, but he trusts his physician enough to agree to the referral. His feelings are ambiguous. He knows that whatever the pain clinic is, it is going to cost him more money; it may turn out like everything else in the past and not work. But he also feels some optimism. Perhaps this is what he needs. Perhaps this pain clinic will be the answer. Perhaps, he can start enjoying life again. Perhaps . . . . Perhaps.

THE PAIN CLINIC

What is a pain clinic? The one to which Mr Jones is being referred is a multidisciplinary setting that will only accept him for treatment after he has been *screened* and *evaluated*. The waiting list for some clinics can be as long as three years (Finer, 1982). Even if he tolerates the waiting, there is a chance that he will not meet the clinic's criteria. If this occurs, he will be referred back to his physician with the reasons for his rejection.

But if he meets the criteria established for the *screening* and *evaluation* phases, he will enter the *treatment* phase. As an inpatient or outpatient, he will work closely with a team of specialists who will follow him through treatment and from one to three years after discharge.

There are other types of pain clinics in existence. They can range from the one-man operation of a chiropractor or acupuncturist, to a clinic that only treats patients with pain from cancer. Because there are presently no firm guidelines for the operation, management and structure of a pain clinic, physicians would do well to know in advance what the different clinics óffer before referring patients to them.

It is estimated that there are over 1000 pain clinics or pain centers now in existence (Casano, 1981). A physicians' referral directory of comprehensive U.S. pain clinics listing a geographic sampling of major centers is available from *Medical World News* (Address: Physicians Referral Directory).

The need for the pain clinic is very clear. National Institutes of Health in the United States published the figure that 15 000 000 adults now have low back pain alone. This results in $5 000 000 for health care costs and 93 000 000 days lost from work. Add to this figure all the other patients who have chronic pain in other sites. Estimates are that one third of the U.S. population has chronic pain, 700 000 000 workdays are lost, and $60 000 000 000 a year are spent in health care costs (Bonica, 1981). Chronic pain is not considered to be a symptom of disease, but rather a disease in itself, says Sternbach (1981).

The team approach

The unique feature of the pain clinic is the interaction that goes on between the patient and health professionals. The patient and the health professionals form a team which will systematically organize and implement tasks with one primary goal: *success*. Who would refute such a goal? No one, but the difficulty that frequently arises is the patient's misunderstanding of the definition of success. To the health professionals on the team, success means effectively guiding the patient into gaining control of his life and chronic pain.

To the patient, success means total eradication of his pain. The most common assumption the patient makes is that he will find someone who can 'fix' his problem. This is a logical assumption and in the U.S.A. our health care system reinforces the concept. The chronic pain patient remains content in his passive health role until it dawns on him that everything he has been told to do and everything that has been done to him has failed. Once he realizes that the traditional approach to health care has failed for him, he becomes receptive to the pain clinic's philosophy. He is ready to assume responsibility for himself under the structured guidance of excellent teachers.

The patient will be taught theories and rationales of pain and also learn various techniques which must be integrated into his daily routine for the rest of his life. This necessary integration is going

to be very difficult after five, ten or fifteen years of a daily routine
of pain behavior. For instance, if the patient cries, takes drugs, yells
at the children, locks himself in the bedroom, or drinks alcoholic
beverages whenever his pain gets unbearable, it will be difficult to
change his conditioned response to pain. There are thousands of
ways he can cope with pain. But all too often these methods are
destructive.

Before going on, let us examine the characteristics of the patient
with chronic pain and the characteristics of the health professional
who will be working with him.

The patient

SHAFT is a mnemonic word often used to describe the chronic
pain patient. It means the Sad, Hostile, Anxious, Frustrated patient
who Tenaciously clings to the health care system (Black, 1975).
This definition appears to be true. It is a very negative statement
about people who are doing what the health care system taught
them to do. The irony is that the system is the failure, not the
patient.

The patient with chronic pain is one of the most misunderstood
patients with whom a health professional will ever work. What hap-
pens to the pain patient in the health care system is disheartening
and often unbelievable, although the pattern and changes are
predictable.

It usually begins with some initial trauma to the body. The patient is physically hurt in some way, and the body's systems are all
alerted to respond as needed. The initial phase of the healing process is called the acute stage and does not last very long. Its duration is usually up to two months, or as long as it takes for the
damaged structure or structures to heal.

After the normal time for tissue healing has passed, the patient
may still have some symptoms of his injury. This period is termed
the subacute stage; it can last from two to six months.

The chronic stage follows the subacute stage and can linger in-
definitely. During this stage, the pain is the one remaining re-
minder of the initial injury. However, all damaged structures are
healed now. The pain is not functioning as it did during the acute
stage when it signaled tissue damage. The chronic pain now has no
real function. Unhappy with continuing pain, the patient becomes
irritable and frustrated. He turns first to his physician for help with
his problem.

'Because the complaint is incompletely understood, many physicians treat chronic pain by using treatments that are effective in acute pain, such as the powerful narcotics and sedative hypnotics. When these drugs are used in chronic pain they rarely, if ever, resolve the pain problem, and they bring with them a host of complications'. (Murphy, 1982)

Not finding the relief from pain that he had hoped for, the patient begins doctor-shopping. The patient does not understand why relieving his pain is such a difficult task. His home pharmacy begins to grow, and he consumes quantities of medications daily. Drug addiction and dependency are common problems.

Besides medications, the patient often will find a physician who offers surgery as another possible pain control measure. These procedures usually fail because many of them are done in the presence of questionable physical evidence. It is generally a futile attempt at 'cutting out' the patient's pain. The chronic pain patient is at 'high risk for iatrogenic complications at the hands of well-meaning physicians.' (Black, 1975)

Patients are commonly referred to physical therapists for massage, ultrasound, hot packs, and exercise. Often, the patient experiences dramatic relief of pain initially. However, these results are temporary. Electroacupressure, electrical stimulation in the form of transcutaneous electrical nerve stimulators, lasers, diathermy and many other physical modalities also are used by physical therapists, but pain relief does not last.

With conventional medical treatments not helping, the patient turns to non-medical personnel and tries almost any possible treatment. He visits chiropractors, reflexologists, acupuncturists, rolfers, etc. Each of these specialists have skills which could benefit the individual with common, uncomplicated pain problems but the chronic pain patient often shows no response to these treatments. How long can someone tolerate a constantly nagging pain before his personality begins to show changes? It is like driving your car with the brakes on, eventually the system wears down. The pain becomes the center of his thoughts. Interactions with family and friends become curtailed because of the fear of the pain worsening. The patient cannot continue his job. He is becoming financially depleted. His whole life seems to be crumbling around him.

His daily routine becomes one of taking medications and staying at home in bed or sitting on a recliner. He has eliminated activity from his routine because every time he attempts an activity his pain level increases.

The patients with chronic pain who have taken the Minnesota Multiphasic Personality Inventory (MMPI) have elevated scores in the part of the test called the 'neurotic triad'. This implies that the patients show patterns of hysteria, hypochondriasis, and depression (Watson, 1982). Between 25 to 65% of the patients are depressed (Kramlinger et al, 1983).

So the patient whose pain started out with the normal, acute response has begun a long unsuccessful search for relief. He has no self-respect or self-confidence left; his depression combined with repetitive failures have led him to despair, making him a high risk for suicide (Finer, 1982). His family and friends are changing in their interactions with the patient. The new distance between them reinforces his feelings of not being loved. Residual organic causes of the pain are now intricately combined with emotional and environmental components. This no longer is called 'just' chronic pain. It is the chronic pain syndrome (Florence, 1981).

'Pain estimate' model

Brena and Koch (1975) projected a 'pain estimate' model to facilitate the quantification and classification of patients with chronic pain syndrome. They took into consideration two variables: (1) the pain behavior (B) or psychological component of the pain resulting from conditioned responses to numerous variables, e.g., emotions, drugs, environment, etc, and (2) the tissue pathology (P) or physical component of the pain.

The pain behavior component of the person's pain was determined by information attained from (1) a semantic inventory (a list of words describing pain), (2) an activity checklist, (3) a drug use rating scale and (4) the MMPI. The pathological component was determined through (1) a physical examination, (2) neurologic testing, (3) laboratory studies and (4) radiology studies. The results of all these tests (Fig. 10.1) were reviewed to give these four classes:

Class 1 patients (p-B) have little or no physical component. All pathology testing gives ambivalent information. They have an increased psychological component evidenced by much pain verbalization, low activity levels, drug abuse and an abnormal MMPI showing personality disturbances. The result is a patient whose pain complaints are verbalized more than any other class, and are commonly called the 'pain amplifiers'.

Class 2 patients (p-b) have little or no physical component, and have little psychological component. Behavior testing shows high

	Behaviour testing				Pathology testing			
	Semantic Inventory	Activity Check-list	Drug-use Rating	M.M.P.I.	Physical Examination	Neurological Testing	Laboratory Studies	Radiology Studies
Class I p-B	High	Low	High	Abnormal	Ambivalent	Ambivalent	Ambivalent	Ambilvalent
Class II p-b	High	Average	Low	Abnormal	Ambivalent	Negative	Negative	Negative
Class III P-B	High	Low	High	Random	Positive	Positive	Positive	Positive
Class IV P-b	Low	High or Average	Low	Random	Positive	Positive	Positive	Positive

*Based on 100 "Pain Estimates" at the Emory Pain Clinic — July–October, 1974 (Work in progress)

Fig. 10.1 Chronic pain states classification (reproduced by permission of Steven F. Brena, 8-2-83).

levels of pain verbalization, average activity levels, little use of medications, and an abnormal MMPI. These patients are the chronic, continuous complainers, the 'pain verbalizers'.

These first two classes of patients described would not benefit from a treatment program focused upon their body (e.g. surgery, nerve blocks and drugs) because there is little or no physical component to their pain. The recommended therapeutic approach would need to emphasize the psychological intervention methods. And, for the class 1 patients, a drug management program is necessary because of their drug abuse problem.

Class 3 patients (P-B) have a high physical (pathological) component confirmed with positive results in all testing procedures; and a high psychological component similar to class 1. This patient has evidence of high levels of both mind and body involvement. Treatments combining physical and psychological strategies equally are required for these 'chronic sufferers'.

Class 4 patients (P-b) also have a high physical component (as did class 3); but a low psychological component. They commonly suffer in silence or de-emphasize their suffering when asked about it. They have high or average activity levels, low intakes of drugs and a random MMPI. Due to the evident physical, pathological findings, removal of the pathological process is the recommended course of action. It is uncommon to see this type of patient referred to a Pain Clinic.

It is obvious that unless the patient has been properly evaluated and diagnosed, it will be impossible to efficiently manage his pain. When the extent of the chronic pain syndrome components are clarified, the appropriate treatment route emerges.

The rest of the team

The health professionals who will work with the chronic pain patient must have comprehensive insights into the nature of this patient, as well as certain attributes which will facilitate interactions with the patient. They must be:
1. skillful and current in their own respective disciplines.
2. dedicated and fully committed to what they are doing.
3. aware of themselves and open to the patient and his unique problems. This self-awareness or sense of self will permit the professionals to handle each situation with integrity, maturity, and forethought.

4. adept in communication from the basic observation and listening skills to the problem solving, counseling and empathy skills.
5. able to simplify concepts so they can be grasped by the patient.
6. patient and creative so they can repeat and/or restate directions and explanations as often as is necessary to facilitate learning in the patient.
7. able to gain the patient's trust, and instill hope in him so that he can learn techniques to control his pain (Thompson, 1981).

Because of the overt humanitarian skills needed, selection of the team members is not usually an easy task. Our pain clinic at the University of Mississippi Medical Center began six years ago as a study group between two professionals (a psychologist and a physical therapist, myself). We expanded by inviting various hand-selected professionals to join us. Before extending the invitations. however, we confirmed that the attributes desired were evident in the individuals (Schaefer & Sturgis, 1982).

Pain clinic teams usually include physicians, psychologists, physical therapists, occupational therapists, recreational therapists, vocational rehabilitation councelors, social workers and nurses. We had a staff which included a dentist, two neurologists, one neuro-surgeon, nurses, two orthopedic surgeons, one physical therapist (the associate director), one psychologist (the director), one respiratory therapist and a psychology resident.

Though it would be ideal to have each of these disciplines represented, I think that the 'basic three' are the core of the team: the physician, the psychologist and the physical therapist. The physician assesses the body's structures and determines the physical, pathological component of his pain; the psychologist assesses the patient's personality and behavior patterns, and determines the extent of the psychological component of his pain; and the physical therapist determines the extent of the body's debilitation from the physical and psychological stresses it has experienced for months, or years.

THE PAIN CLINIC PROCESS

There are four main phases in the pain clinic's procedure. Each phase hinges on the one chronologically before it. The phases are: *screening, evaluation, treatment,* and *follow-up.*

Screenings

Most patients have a long wait before they are scheduled to be seen

for screening. The functions of this intitial meeting are to:
1. confirm that the patient is an appropriate candidate for the clinics, and
2. familiarize the patient with the approach that would be used in the clinic. He must understand the whole picture of treatment so he can decide if he is ready for the commitment and hard work.

We use the following criteria:

1. *Litigation.* If a patient is involved in litigation, or if litigation is pending, he is not accepted. If the patient is involved in financial matters concerning his pain state, he can often be distracted from his task at hand which is working hard with the health professionals on the pain clinic team. (Some clinics will accept patients who are pending litigation.) (Chapman et al, 1981)

2. *Pain lasting longer than six months.* There are a few pain clinics which accept patients during the subacute stage (three to six months); however, the majority require a minimum of six months duration before consideration is given for their admission. This duration criterion insures that the structures originally injured have healed adequately.

3. *Cancer.* Patients with cancer are not accepted to our clinic.

4. *Physician referral.* This is a universal given for pain clinics. The patient must be referred by a physician, who agrees to forward all medical records. The physician must also agree to follow the patient after discharge, when necessary.

5. *Family participation.* The family must agree to participate. The family's role often is overlooked in the treatment of the pain patient. However, family members may be part of the patient's pain problem. How they view the person in pain, how much they understand the pain process, how they deal with the negative pain behaviors they see, how they contribute to the person's pain, and what they can do to facilitate the person's improvement are but a small sample of the topics to be explored.

6. *Motivation.* The patient has to want to get better and also be committed to putting the time and energy into this endeavor. He must be ready to take responsibility for his health and the management of his pain. He must be open to learning and practicing the skills he will be taught. Sometimes the skills taught appear to be so simple that the patient underestimates their value.

7. *Conceptual understanding.* With the patient anxious to be helped, and happy to finally be given an appointment with a pain clinic representative, it is very possible that he will not hear everything being said or that items will be misconstrued and misunder-

stood. When he leaves this initial meeting he must understand that the clinic is not a fast fix-it, and if he is accepted, he and his family have a lot of hard work ahead.

If the patient makes it past the *screening*, he will then be scheduled for the next phase: *evaluation*. In the interim, he is started on record keeping and given supplemental information to read about the clinic.

8. *Record keeping.* The patient is directed to fill out daily activity records (DAR) which are divided into hourly increments over each 24 hour period. The DAR requests information on: time spent out of the reclining or sitting position (up-time), time spent reclining or sitting (down-time), pain level (numerical value on a scale from 0–10), mood, medications, and a short description of his activities.

This is just the beginning of his record keeping for the patient who continues through the total program. Record keeping is very important in determining the patient's compliance and in establishing baseline values on each item for use in comparative data. The patient is advised to bring his completed records and all this medications to the evaluation.

Evaluation

The evaluation phase is the most important part of the pain clinic progression. A thorough evaluation from the appropriate team members will save a lot of time in determining the proper treatment. It may be done as an inpatient or as an outpatient. Not all team members will be involved with every patient. Those who will be evaluating the patient will be notified after the initial screening.

1. Physicians. Orthopedists, neurologists, neurosurgeons, psychiatrists, physiatrists, anesthesiologists, and internists can all be associated with the clinic, and contacted for consultation. The specific medical evaluation(s) needed is/are determined by the problem(s) the patient presents.

Tests will be ordered as needed: x-rays, computerized axial tomography (CAT-scans), electromyograms (EMG), nerve conduction velocities (NCV), thermograms (Scott & Huskisson, 1976), etc. A good history is taken. The old records are reviewed and integrated with the new findings. The musculoskeletal system is astutely evaluated along with all the medications that the patient is taking.

The physician's tasks are to identify specific structural problems and to substantiate organic components for the pain. These tasks are very difficult, but are compounded when the patient arrives at the pain clinic with multiple diagnoses from all his former physicians. These previous diagnoses should not be accepted readily but substantiated or eliminated by the Pain Clinic physician.

2. *Psychologist.* This evaluation will usually be two-fold: a pen-and-paper portion and a personal interview.

Pen-and-paper. Two of the most common tests given today in Pain Clinics are the MMPI and the MMPQ (the Melzack McGill Pain Questionnaire). Both tests have proven to be valid and reliable in gathering information on the chronic pain patient. These tests, when properly scored and interpreted, can identify personality and learning factors that maintain the pain behavior (Cox et al, 1978; Melzack, 1975).

The MMPI consists of 566 statements on a variety of topics: physical condition, moral attitudes, social behavior, personal characteristics, etc. The patient assesses each of the statements as true or false as applied to himself (Cohen et al, 1983). The results, which can be computer analyzed, yield four validity scales and 10 basic clinical or personality scales.

The MMPQ focuses upon gathering data about the properties of the patient's pain experience. It is usually administered by a research assistant, who ensures that the patient understands what is being asked. There are several components to this test. However, it primarily consists of word descriptors which the patient uses to describe his subjective pain experience. These words are divided into three major classes: sensory, affective and evaluative (Fig. 10.2).

The interview. Patients are probably the most hesitant when it comes to this evaluation. They may have been told: 'it is all in your head. You need to see a psychiatrist.' The patient's interpretation of this comment is that someone thinks his pain is imaginary. The stigma of seeing a psychiatrist or psychologist is still strong in Western society.

For this reason, the psychologist's task may be initially more difficult than any other team member. The goal, however, is to integrate the information from past medical records with the new information about the patient's behavior, personality, family, and mechanism of secondary gain. The Daily Activity Records are reviewed and clarified especially those areas related to the patient's mood and pain perception ratings.

3. *Physical therapist.* This evaluation can determine the extent to which psychological and structural forces have debilitated the body. The emphasis is placed upon the patient's functional capabilities.

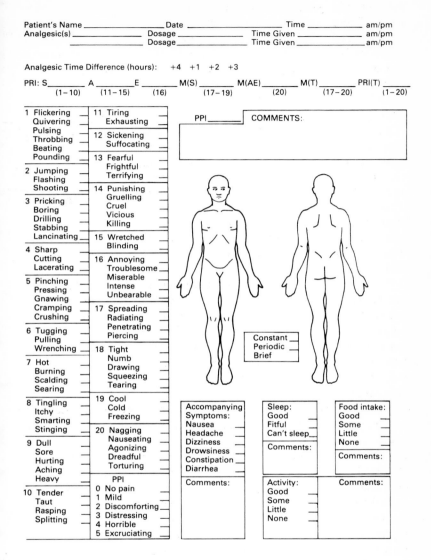

Patient's Name _____ Date _____ Time _____ am/pm
Analgesic(s) _____ Dosage _____ Time Given _____ am/pm
                  _____ Dosage_____ Time Given _____ am/pm

Analgesic Time Difference (hours):   +4 +1 +2 +3

PRI: S_____ A _____E _____ M(S) _____ M(AE)_____ M(T) _____ PRI(T) _____
        (1–10)   (11–15)   (16)   (17–19)   (20)   (17–20)   (1–20)

1 Flickering
  Quivering
  Pulsing
  Throbbing
  Beating
  Pounding
	11 Tiring
	  Exhausting
	12 Sickening
	  Suffocating
	13 Fearful
	  Frightful
	  Terrifying
		PPI_____ COMMENTS:

2 Jumping
  Flashing
  Shooting		

3 Pricking
  Boring
  Drilling
  Stabbing
  Lancinating
	14 Punishing
	  Gruelling
	  Cruel
	  Vicious
	  Killing	

4 Sharp
  Cutting
  Lacerating
	15 Wretched
	  Blinding
	16 Annoying
	  Troublesome
	  Miserable
	  Intense
	  Unbearable	

5 Pinching
  Pressing
  Gnawing
  Cramping
  Crushing
	17 Spreading
	  Radiating
	  Penetrating
	  Piercing	

6 Tugging
  Pulling
  Wrenching
	18 Tight
	  Numb
	  Drawing
	  Squeezing
	  Tearing
		Constant
		Periodic
		Brief

7 Hot
  Burning
  Scalding
  Searing
	19 Cool
	  Cold
	  Freezing	

8 Tingling
  Itchy
  Smarting
  Stinging
	20 Nagging
	  Nauseating
	  Agonizing
	  Dreadful
	  Torturing
		Accompanying
		Symptoms:
		Nausea
		Headache
		Dizziness
		Drowsiness
		Constipation
		Diarrhea
			Sleep:
			Good
			Fitful
			Can't sleep
			Comments:
				Food intake:
				Good
				Some
				Little
				None
				Comments:

9 Dull
  Sore
  Hurting
  Aching
  Heavy				

10 Tender
  Taut
  Rasping
  Splitting
	PPI
	0 No pain
	1 Mild
	2 Discomforting
	3 Distressing
	4 Horrible
	5 Excruciating
		Comments:	Activity:
			Good
			Some
			Little
			None
				Comments:

Fig. 10.2 The McGill Melzack Pain Questionnaire. The classes of words are sensory, 1 to 10; affective, 11 to 15; evaluative, 16; and miscellaneous; 17 to 20. The rank value of each word is based on the position in the word set. The sum of the rank values is the pain rating index (PRI). The index of the present pain intensity (PPI) is based on a scale of 0 to 5. (copyright R. Melzack, 1970) Reproduced by permission of R. Melzack, 8-4-83.

The initial evaluations of strength, flexibility, endurance, joint play and sensation are coupled with evaluations of static and dynamic alignment and palpation to locate trigger points or isolated points of tenderness. On occasion, photographs are taken to document a specific problem for later comparisons.

The results of these tests and the information on the daily activity records concerning activities, up-time, down-time and pain level, are integrated with the past medical records.

4. *Nurses.* Information on bowel problems, medications, food allergies, nutrition, smoking, caffeine intake, sleep problems and self-care problems are accumulated.

5. *Vocational rehabilitation counselor.* The patient's work history and work goals are obtained. The counselor will attempt to find out if there are more reasons for the patient to stay in pain than for him to give it up. In the U.S.A., society tends to pay people to be sick, and this financial compensation sometimes inhibits work recovery. Thus, if it appears feasible, a well-organized work-directed program will be needed.

6. *Occupational therapist.* The performance of the normal activities of daily living will be assessed. All too often, treatment goals get set without having a complete understanding of the patient's functional limitations, e.g. combing his hair, putting on a pull-over sweater, getting in and out of a car, picking up his six-month-old baby, putting on his socks or getting in and out of a bath tub. Unless each of these problems is addressed, the patient will not be able to address other, more complex problems.

7. *Recreational therapist.* Information is gathered on the patient's present use of leisure time and his interests in sports, reading or other hobbies.

8. *Respiratory therapist.* The patient's lung volumes are recorded and will be compared to future lung volumes. Many of our chronic pain patients are unable to breathe regularly during activities of daily living. Often they display a tendency to hold their breath.

After all the evaluations have been completed, a special meeting of the evaluators is called. Each of us values this face-to-face interaction for two reasons. First, it shows that we respect each other by making time to be present. Second, this is a period of open communication and sharing among the team. We discuss the results of our evaluations and integrate them into a whole picture. (In most cases, the patient has been informed of our individual evaluation results as we did the testing.)

To graphically document the evaluation results and provide a visual reference to this baseline information, the Patient Evaluation Conference System (PECS) was devised by Harvey and Jellinek. This computerized technique displays the assessment results in bar graph form. The patient profile is divided into 15 categories (Fig. 10.3) which relate to the patient's functional abilities. The usefulness of the PECS is evident also during the treatment phase of the program. Functional improvements are easily added to the initial visual scale.

Our next step is to discuss the integrated summary and recommendations with the patient. It is at this point that the patient usually decides to continue in the program and begin the treatment phase with the other team members, withdraw from the program totally, or temporarily delay the beginning of the treatment phase.

Treatment

Treatment programs can be conducted on an inpatient or outpatient basis. Inpatient stays vary between clinics from two to eight weeks. Also the number of available beds varies between clinics, ranging from three to forty-five. Inpatient treatment is the more common trend, especially for patients with evident drug problems. However, this approach has prompted strong opposition from some who believe the patient should not be taken out of his own environment. The inpatient setting is considered to be artificial because the patient is without his normal routine stresses to distract him. After discharge, he is placed back into his home setting.

1. Physician. Medication adjustment and easing drug withdrawal will be primary tasks. During the first few days in the hospital the patient has at his disposal all the medications that he has brought from home. These are kept at the nurses' station. They are readily given when the patient asks and in the quantity requested. A precise record is kept (Black, 1975). It would seem easier to ask the patient what medications he is taking. However, studies have shown that patients generally are inaccurate when giving self-reports on drug usage (Ready et al, 1982).

Once medication levels of the patient are established, the pharmacist devises a pain cocktail or tablet that will be administered on a strict schedule. The scheduling of medications cannot be over-emphasized. It is needed to 'establish and maintain a constant blood plasma drug level' (Atkinson, 1983). In this way the patient has greater relief, takes fewer drugs and does not exceed his threshold of tolerance.

Patient evaluation conference system (PECS) (copyright Harvey and Jellinek, 1979)

Scores range from 0 to 7. with 0 being the lowest score or not assessed. and 7 being the highest score, such as normal or independent. Scores of 1 to 4 indicate dependent function. Scores of 5 or more indicate independent function.

I. Rehabilitation Medicine (MED)
1. Motor loss
2. Spasticity/involuntary movem't
3. Joint limitations
4. Autonomic disturbance
5. Sensory deficiency
6. Perceptual & cognitive defic'cy
7. Associated medical problems

II. Rehabilitation Nursing (NSG)
1. Performance of bowel program
2. Performance of urinary program
3. Performance of skin program
4. Assume respons. for self-care
5. Perf. assigned int'disc. activ.

III· Physical Mobility (PHY)
1. Performance of transfers
2. Performance of ambulation
3. Performance of w/c mobility
4. Abil. to handle environ.barriers
5. Performance of car transfer
6. Driving mobility
7. Assumes respons. for mobility

IV. Activities of Daily Living (ADL)
1. Performance in feeding
2. Performance in hygiene/grooming
3. Performance in dressing
4. Performance in home management
5. Perf. of mobility — home environ.

V. Communication (COM)
1. Comprehend spoken language
2. Produce language
3. Read
4. Produce written language
5. Hear
6. Comprehend & use gesture
7. Produce speech

VI. Medications (DRG)
1. Knowledge of medications
2. Skill with medications
3. Utilization of medications

VII. Nutrition (NUT)
1. Nutritional status — body weight
2. Nutritional status — lab. values
3. Knowledge of nutrition &/or diet
4. Skill with nutrition &/or diet
5. Utilization of nutrition & diet

VIII. Assistive Devices (DEV)
1. Knowledge of assistive device(s)
2. Skill with assuming operating position of assistive device(s)
3. Utilization of assistive device(s)

IX. Psychology (PSY)
1. Distress/comfort
2. Helplessnesss/self-efficacy
3. Self-directed learning skills
4. Skill in self-management of behavior and emotions
5. Skill in interpersonal relations

X. Neuropsychology (NP)
1. Impairment — short-term memory
2. Impairment — long-term memory
3. Impair. — att'n/concen. skills
4. Impair. — verbal linguistic processing
5. Impair. — visual spatial processing
6. Impair. — basic intellectual skills

XI. Social Issues (SOC)
1. Ability to problem solve and utilize resources
2. Family: communication/resource
3. Family: understand disability
4. Economic resources
5. Ability to live independently
6. Living arrangements

XII. Vocat'l/Educat'l Activity (V/E)
1. Active participation in realistic voc/ed planning
2. Realistic perception of work-related activity
3. Abil. to tolerate planned no. of hrs of voc/ed activity per day
4. Voc/ed placement
5. Physical capacity for work

XIII. Recreation (REC)
1. Particip. in group activities
2. Particip. in community activ.
3. Interaction with others
4. Participation & satisfaction w/individual leisure activities
5. Active participation in sports

XIV. Pain (concensus) (PAI)
1. Pain behavior
2. Physical inactivity
3. Social withdrawal
4. Pacing
5. Sitting tolerance
6. Standing tolerance
7. Walking tolerance

XV. Pulmonary Rehabilitation (PUL)
1. Knowledge of pulm. rehab. prog.
2. Skill with pulm. rehab. prog.
3. Utiliz. of pulm. rehab. prog.

Fig. 10.3 Key to functional ability item abbreviations used with the profile.

The medication schedule also eliminates many of the patient's anxieties. For instance, he does not have to ask the nurse for his medications and face possible intimidation (real or perceived). Any guilt feelings about taking too many or narcotic-type medications are alleviated. He also is aware that his pain tolerance level will probably not be reached on this regular schedule. Medications are taken out of his control, so they can become de-emphasized in their role of pain relief.

The medication will be gradually reduced. Though the patient knows that this is going to be done, he is not overtly aware of when the decreases occur because the cocktail or tablet continues to look the same. As the medications are being reduced, they are being replaced with other nonchemical methods of pain control, taught by other team members.

Besides easing withdrawal from addictive drugs, the physician will substitute (interchange) the drugs. Too frequently the patient is on drugs that treat acute pain very efficiently, but only serve to increase chronic pain (Black, 1975; Bonica, 1981; Murphy 1982; Turner et al, 1982).

2. Psychologist. Because of the tendency toward the 'neurotic triad', the psychologist's treatments emphasize methods to reduce anxiety, depression, hypochondriasis, and hysteria. Hypnosis, bio-feedback (electromyographic (EMG), Galvanic Skin Response (GSR) and thermal) and relaxation training are commonly used.

The patient is guided into problem-solving techniques, assertiveness training, strategies for efficient utilization and management of time, goal setting, pacing, and stress management skills. Counselling sessions involve the patient and his family. Mutual problem areas are discussed (e.g. sexual, social, etc).

Throughout all of this, a common theme surfaces: pain has a psychological component that can be controlled. After this basic premise is understood and the patient understands 'why this happened,' progress becomes evident. All healthy behaviors are reinforced (behavior modification), while the unhealthy behaviors are de-emphasized or ignored.

3. *Physical therapist.* The treatment focuses upon decreasing pain symptomology and increasing function. A progressive exercise program, tailored to the patient, is established. This will emphasize strengthening weakened muscles, lengthening shortened muscles and increasing general endurance. The specific numerical results of this exercise program will be charted and used to give feedback to the patient. In order to progress the patient maximally, specific daily quotas are set for the patient, and the patient is aware of these goals (Doleys et al, 1982).

Mobilization is done if necessary to restore accessory motion to the joint. Pain and the accompanying trigger or tender areas can be treated in a variety of ways: ice massage (Aronoff, 1982a); traditional massage; acupressure; electrical stimulation in the form of Transcutaneous Electrical Nerve Stimulation (TENS) (Frampton, 1982), electroacupressure, or high voltage stimulation; ultrasound; superficial heat; cold; and traction, manual or mechanical. The patient is taught proper body mechanics for lifting, reaching, sitting and bending. The whole staff reinforces these throughout his treatment and especially during his exercise program. The importance of proper breathing during movement is taught along with the relationship of relaxation to breathing (Schaefer, 1983).

The patient is given nightly assignments to maintain his program and guide him to an increased awareness of his body's signal system. Continuous practice of his pain control strategies is essential.

4. *Nurses.* When the patient is back on the ward after a full day of scheduled activities, he often finds himself with nothing to do. Such inactivity can make him slip back into his old, conditioned pain behaviors, e.g., sitting in a slouched position while watching television; worrying about problems over which he has no control; drinking caffeine and smoking excessively; complaining to a friend on the phone; requesting extra medications, etc. The nurse must be able to recognize these behaviors for what they are and diplomatically guide the patient through the strategies that he has

learned so he can regain control of his situation. How successful a patient is at managing his free time on the ward is a crucial insight into how successful he will be at home. The ward and the home are intimately linked.

5. *Social worker.* A close working relationship between the psychologist and the social worker is necessary; together they identify and attempt to resolve with the patient the problems facing him and his family.

6. *Occupational therapist.* The O.T. instructs the patient in easier, more efficient methods of performing activities of daily living. The patient is made aware of numerous self-help devices. If the patient is preparing to go back to work, job-related activities are planned. These activities parallel the physical therapy program. They build endurance to work-related tasks.

7. *Recreational therapist.* This health professional establishes programs which will guide the use of 'free' time into activities—usually hobby related—that the patient enjoys.

8. *Respiratory therapist.* In our pain clinic the respiratory therapist does pulmonary testing, and works closely with the physical therapist on exercises to improve poor breathing habits.

All activities during the patient's treatment phase are scheduled in advance, so the patient knows where he needs to be at specific times. He is responsible for maintaining this schedule. This strategy of advanced scheduling is used for many reasons. First, the patient has the example set for continued productivity after discharge. Second, he is becoming disciplined to activity after weeks, months or years of little or no activity. Third, the importance of pacing the activities is constantly reinforced by the scheduled periods of rest and skill-practicing sessions. And finally, the patient realizes that he can increase his activities without an increase in pain if he remains aware of his body and handles any symptom at the time it appears.

At Rancho Los Amigos in California, the daily performance levels and up-time of the patient are recorded on a graphic display measuring two feet by three feet (Cairns et al, 1976). This display is located above the patient's bed and provides a guideline for the staff concerning the appropriate behavior modification responses that should be used. Praise and attention from the staff are used if improvement is reflected. Negative pain behaviors are not reinforced.

Discharge

By the time of discharge, the patient should have learned the strategies for handling pain. Pain levels have decreased since the day of admission. If physical changes were necessary in the home (rearrangement of furniture, the purchase of a step stool, a firmer mattress, hand grips on the wall to assist getting into and out of the bath tub, etc.), they have been completed by now. If the patient has prepared to go back to work, then he is scheduled to return the Monday after his Friday discharge.

The patient is given the clinic phone numbers in case problems arise. However, by this time the patient recognizes that the responsibility for his continued health success falls on his shoulders. He is unlikely to ever be abused by the health care system again because he now knows and understands the role of the health professionals as well as his role in his own health care. Clinic personnel will usually call the patient once a week initially to ensure continued success.

In addition to regular initial phone contact, return visits are scheduled. We see the patient once a week for the first month, then once a month for three months, and once every six months for the remainder of a three-year span.

Follow-up

These scheduled follow-up visits are not to be taken lightly. They are as important as all other components of the pain clinic progression. Now back in his own environment, the patient is battling against his old routine. Even with the help of a supportive family and newly learned skills, this adjustment to home is not easy.

The patient continues to keep daily activity records as long as it is feasible. They are brought to the follow-up visits and reviewed. Family members usually come with the patient initially so that unanticipated problems can be resolved early.

Sometimes it becomes necessary for a patient to be re-admitted for a short, intensive refresher course. But this re-admission can often be averted by the patient's active participation in support groups. The function of these groups is similar to Alcoholic Anonymous and Over-eaters Anonymous. Aronoff has started a support group in Boston called the 'Pain Copers'.

EFFECTIVENESS

How effective are the pain clinics? This is a hard question to answer because there are so many variables. How do you measure the patient's perception of pain? Can one patient with chronic pain be validly compared to someone else in chronic pain? Can pain clinics be compared when their approaches are different? How do you measure success? These and other questions have been raised by many authors reporting follow-up information on their clinics (Aronoff et al, 1983; Aronoff, 1982b; Hallett & Pilowsky, 1982; Sturgis et al, 1984).

The most common questions concerning the effectiveness or success of the pain clinic methods are discussed here.

Question one: How do you measure the patient's perception of pain?

Pain is a subjective personal experience, with no two people responding exactly the same way to a constant painful stimulus. To attempt measurement of this subjective experience, an objective tool must be used. Two methods are described here, the numerical system and the visual analogue scale (VAS).

Numerical system. Two common numerical scales are used: 0 to 100 and 0 to 10. In each case, the zero means 'no pain' and the other extreme numerical end of the scale means 'excruciating pain'. The patient is asked to rate his pain by giving it a numerical value.

Visual analogue scale (VAS). The VAS is a vertical or horizontal line drawing, usually 10 cm long with extreme ends clearly defined. Each end has a descriptor that takes the scale from 'no pain' to 'maximum, excruciating pain'. The patient is directed to mark the scale at the point that would reflect his pain level. A ruler placed along the scale is used to translate the information into a numerical value. These scales are only valid for statistical manipulation when the patient completes each without reference to his previous estimates (Scott & Huskisson, 1976).

Question two: Can pain clinics be compared?

Treatments in a pain clinic should not be identical for each patient. Treatments in one pain clinic will not be identical to the treatments in another. Comparisons of results obtained thus may be difficult to make. As previously pointed out, pain clinics differ greatly.

Some are inpatient facilities; others are in outpatient settings. Some have a large number of health professionals working as a collaborative team, others have few health professionals. Some clinics emphasize the behavioral, psychological component of the patient's treatment; others emphasize the physical components; and still others blend the two approaches in their treatment protocols.

Question three: How do you measure success?

In addition to the patient's quantified pain rating, the most common measures used to document progress in one pain clinic's patient population are: (1) up time changes; (2) drug intake changes; (3) employment status; (4) changes on the MMPI; and (5) changes in physical function.

 1. *Up-time.* If the patient stays on his feet for longer periods than he did upon his initial admission, then improvement is usually assumed. To take just one measurement of patient improvement without consideration for the other related areas would be incomplete. Often, up-time changes are correlated with the patient's pain rating.

 Sanders has devised a method to document precisely the amount of time a patient spends in an upright position. The patient carries a miniature electronic stopwatch that has a mercury-tilt trigger mounted on the patient's thigh. Whenever the patient is standing, the trigger activates the stopwatch, and up-time is precisely accumulated. Studies comparing the use of this devise to subjects recording their own up-time showed there is a tendency for self-reports to be lower than actual up-time (Sanders, 1983; Sanders, 1980).

 2. *Drugs.* Comparisons of drug quantities and drug types are documented. The ideal trend would show a decrease in narcotic medications accompanied by a temporary increase in non-narcotic medications. When the patient's pain is stabilized, another decrease in the quantity of non-narcotic medication would occur.

 Similar to up-time documentation, reports of medication changes alone would be inconclusive. But, if drug changes were coupled with the patient's pain ratings or up-time changes, the reports would be useful.

 3. *Employment status.* If a patient has been unable to work because of pain, then his return to work often symbolizes success. However, you cannot omit information on the quality of his work, the type of work (the same or different), the number of hours a day

worked now compared to before, the patient's pain levels and/or medication intake. All of this information is pertinent to his 'going back to work'.

I personally believe that success is not necessarily measured by employment status in the U.S.A. Too many factors enter into a person's ability to gain employment in these times. Jobs may not be available; the patient may not need the money; the patient may be too old or not as competitive as others because he has been away from the work setting for a relatively long period of time; and, of course, employers may be hesitant to hire anyone with a 'disability'.

4. *MMPI*. The scores on the MMPI are initially high on the hysteria, hypochondriasis and depression scales for the patient with chronic pain. As the patient's pain decreases, these scores also are known to decrease into normal ranges.

5. *Function*. Upon admission to a pain clinic, the patient displays little tolerance to physical activity. During physical therapy, occupational therapy and recreational therapy sessions there is documentation of all exercise progressions, strength changes, flexibility changes, and endurance increases. These records can very clearly quantify the increase in the patient's activity level. This information coupled with the patient's pain ratings and medication intake can substantiate the patient's improvement.

Question four: When and how should data be obtained from the patient after discharge?

During the evaluation and treatment phases of the program the patient begins keeping records. He may continue keeping them even throughout his follow-up visits. These accumulated data can be used to quantify the patient's progress very easily.

But if the data are not available after he has been discharged, there are two questions with which we are faced: how much time should lapse before contacting the patient and how should this information be gathered?

1. *When?* There does not seem to be any trend emerging in the literature to suggest when the 'best' or 'worst' times are for contacting the patient. Initial evaluations have indicated 50–70% of the patients who complete comprehensive treatment programs show maintenance of treatment gains at one to six month follow-up (Aronoff et al, 1983; Cairns et al, 1976; Chapman et al, 1981). But we also need to know if this trend continues. Does the patient continue doing well?

2. How? Most of the information obtained from the patient after discharge is done through questionnaires or telephone contact. Chapman et al (1981) were able to conduct face-to-face interviews. Regardless of the method used, the patient's memory is challenged. This is a problem because the patient's memory concerning past pain is inaccurate (Linton & Melin, 1982).

Just a few of the difficulties encountered in reporting outcomes of the pain clinic have been discussed. There are others such as the failure to use control groups and the inadequate numbers of patients for the studies to show statistical significance. One hopes that some directives will be forthcoming to guide chronic pain researchers into some consistent, valid and reliable methods of collecting data so that the effectiveness of our clinics can be critically reviewed.

CONCLUSION

Over the last six years I have been treating the patient with chronic pain. Initially, it was difficult to organize the pain clinic at the University of Mississippi Medical Center and gain the support of other health professions. But now, after it has been functional, there is little doubt that pain clinics are a necessary entity in our health care system in the U.S.A.

In a way this is very sad because these clinics are often focused on the patients who are the iatrogenic misfortunes or oversights of our present health care system. Acute pain does *not* need to progress to chronic pain; chronic pain does *not* need to progress to the chronic pain syndrome. But to prevent these from occurring, the patient needs better management from astute health professionals and a better understanding of his own body and health.

REFERENCES

Address: Physicians' Referral Directory of Comprehensive U.S. Pain Clinics, Medical World News, 1221 Avenue of the Americas, New York, New York 10020.
Aronoff G M, Evans W O, Enders P L 1983 A review of follow-up studies of multidisciplinary pain units. Pain 16: 1–11.
Aronoff G M 1982a Ice massage for pain. Aches & Pain 3: 33–36.
Aronoff G M 1982b Pain Clinic #2. Pain units provide an effective alternative technique in the management of chronic pain. Orthopaedic Review 11: 95–100.
Atkinson J H 1983 Current perspectives in the management of chronic pain. Drug Therapy (June): 73–88.

Black R G 1975 The chronic pain syndrome. Surgical Clinics of North America 55: 999–1011.

Bonica J J 1981 Editorial. Triangle 20: 1–6.

Brena S F, Koch D L 1975 A "pain estimate" model for quantification and classification of chronic pain states. Anesthesiology Review 2: 8–13.

Cairns D, Thomas L, Pace J B 1976 Comprehensive treatment approach to chronic low back pain. Pain 2: 301–308.

Carlsson A M 1983 Assessment of chronic pain I. Aspects of the reliability and validity of the Visual Analogue Scale. Pain 16: 87–101.

Casano K 1981 Pain Clinics: which one for your patient? Aches & Pains 2: 8–12.

Catchlove R, Cohen K 1982 Effects of a directive return to work approach in the treatment of workman's compensation patients with chronic pain. Pain 14: 181–191.

Chapman S L, Brena S F, Bradford L A 1981 Treatment outcome in a chronic pain rehabilitation program. Pain 11: 255–268.

Cohen C A, Foster H M, Peck E A 1983 MMPI evaluation of patients with chronic pain. Southern Medical Journal 76: 316–321.

Cox G B, Chapman C R, Black R G 1978 The MMPI and chronic pain: the diagnosis of psychogenic pain. Journal of Behavioral Medicine 1: 437–443.

Doleys D M, Crocker M, Patton D 1982 Response of patients with chronic pain to exercise quotas. Physical Therapy 62: 1111–1114.

Finer B 1982 Treatment in an interdisciplinary pain clinic. In Barber, Adrian (eds) Psychological approaches to the management of pain. Bruner/Mazel Inc, New York, ch 11, pp 186–203.

Florence D W 1981 The chronic pain syndrome. A physical and psychologic challenge. Chronic Pain Syndrome 70: 217–228.

Frampton V M 1982 Pain control with the aid of transcutaneous nerve stimulation. Physiotherapy 68: 77–81.

Hallett E C, Pilowsky I 1982 The response to treatment in a multidisciplinary pain clinic. Pain 12: 365–374.

Hammonds W, Brena S F, Unikel I P 1978 Compensation for work-related injuries and rehabilitation of patients with chronic pain. Southern Medical Journal 71: 664–666.

Harvey R F, Jellinek H M 1983 Patient profiles: utilization in functional performance assessment. Archives of Physical Medicine and Rehabilitation 64: 268–271.

Hendler N, Uematsu S, Long D 1982 Thermographic validation of physical complaints in 'psychogenic pain' patients. Psychosomatics 23: 283–287.

Kramlinger K G, Swanson D W, Maruta T 1983 Are patients with chronic pain depressed? American Journal of Psychiatry 140: 747–749.

Linton S J, Melin L 1982 The accuracy of remembering chronic pain. Pain 13: 281–285.

Melzack R 1975 The McGill Pain Questionnaire: major properties and scoring methods. Pain 1: 277–299.

Murphy T 1982 Techniques for the evaluation and treatment of pain. Lesson 9: Use and abuse of drugs in chronic pain states. Surgical Practice News (January): 9–10 (19).

Ready L B, Sarkis E, Turner J A 1982 Self-reported vs. actual use of medications in chronic pain patients. Pain 12: 285–294.

Sanders S H 1983 Automated versus self-monitoring of 'up time' in chronic low-back pain patients: a comparative study. Pain 15: 399–405.

Sanders S H 1980 Toward a practical instrument system for the automatic measurement of 'up-time' in chronic pain patients. Pain 9: 103–109.

Schaefer C A 1983 It only hurts when I breathe. Aches & Pains 4: 52–54.

Schaefer C A, Sturgis E T 1982 Physical Therapy: A prominent component of the

Pain Clinic at the University of Mississippi Medical Center. Proceedings of the World Confederation of Physical Therapists. Stockholm, Sweden, p 506–509.

Scott J, Huskisson E C 1976 Graphic representation of pain. Pain 2: 175–184.

Sternbach R A 1981 Chronic pain as a disease entity. Triangle 20: 27–32.

Sturgis E T, Schaefer C A, Sikora T L 1984 Follow-up study of a pain center: treated and untreated patients. Archives of Physical Medicine and Rehabilitation 65:301–303.

Thompson S C 1981 Will it hurt less if I can control it? A complex answer to a simple question. Psychological Bulletin 90: 89–101.

Turner J A, Calsyn D A, Fordyce W E, Ready L B 1982 Drug utilization patterns in chronic pain patients. Pain 12: 357–363.

Watson D 1982 Neurotic tendencies among chronic pain patients: an MMPI item analysis. Pain 14: 365–385.

CONTENTS

Annotated bibliography

An annotated bibliography in this volume on Pain represents a select set of articles which the authors of these chapters have found particularly helpful to them as they formulated their thoughts for this publication. Many selections are references for clinicians needing specific information as they treat their patients. Other references are more philosophical, or more didactic. It is not meant to be a comprehensive bibliography, but rather a sketch of references which these authors, the editor of this volume, and Peter Wells, a Physical Therapist working at the Royal Free Hospital in London, have found especially timely, relevant, and clinically helpful. They are primarily articles written by physical therapists, published within the past 5 years, and are found in the geographical region where the author is located. The reader will have some basis, we hope, for deciding which articles would be most useful to himself, and whether it would be worthwhile to go to some extraordinary means to obtain the original article. If an article is unobtainable, the annotation may provide enough information to make use of the basic information contained within an article.

PART 1
A. BASIC PAIN MECHANISMS

Basbaum A I, Field H L 1978 Endogenous pain control mechanisms: Review and hypothesis. Annals of Neurology 4: 451.
This provides an excellent review of the current neurophysiologic mechanisms related to electroanalgesia. The authors discuss the transmission of nociceptive information and the nervous system (brainstem) structures that modulate and perhaps liberate neurohumoral substances.

Bishop B 1980 Pain: Its physiology and rationale for management. Part I: Neuroanatomical substrate of pain, pp 13–20. Part II: Analgesic systems of the CNS, pp 21–23. Part III: Consequences of current concepts of pain mechanisms related to pain management, pp 24–27. References, pp 27–37 Physical Therapy 60(1): 13–37.
This three part series, written by a prominent physiologist who has long held an interest in physical therapy, and who wrote the foreword to this book,

presents an unusually complete review of the neurophysiology of pain. A historical perspective is followed by a straightforward anatomical and functional description of pain receptors, neural pathways, and neural transmitters in Part I. Part II discusses endogenous morphine-like substances and the possible use of these in pain control. Part III describes how some treatment approaches (acupuncture and TENS especially), as well as drugs, provide analgesia based on a revised gate-control theory. Of great value is the extensive reference list at the end of the series, arranged topically and related to sections within each of the three parts.

Messing R B, Lytle L D 1977 Serotonin-containing neurons: Their possible role in pain and analgesia. Pain 4: 1.
A comprehensive analysis of serotonin, its synthesis, liberation and function in the pain process is provided.

Wells P E 1982 Cervical dysfunction and shoulder problems. Physiotherapy 68(3): 66–73.
This paper explores the relationship between cervical degenerative change and shoulder symptoms and signs. It is argued that because the true origin of many shoulder problems is not identified as within the cervical spine, their treatment, if directed entirely to the shoulder, is usually unacceptably protracted and finally unsatisfactory. A review is included of investigations which have demonstrated that traumatised vertebral tissues, apart from nerve roots, give rise to patterns of referred pain, tenderness and other phenomena in the shoulder region. The mechanism of such shoulder pain and dysfunction is explored. A group of suitable tests to clarify the degree of cervical involvement is described.

B. EVALUATION OF PAIN

Carlsson A M 1983 Assessment of chronic pain. I. Aspects of the reliability and validity of the Visual Analogue scale. Pain 16: 87–101.
The visual analogue scale (VAS) is a simple and frequently used method for the assessment of variations in intensity of pain. In clinical practice the percentage of pain relief, assessed by the VAS, is often considered as a measure of the efficacy of treatment. However, as illustrated in the present study, the validity of VAS estimates performed by patients with chronic pain may be unsatisfactory. Two types of VAS, an absolute and a comparative scale, were compared with respect to factors influencing the reliability and validity of pain estimates. As shown in this study the absolute type of VAS seems to be less sensitive to bias than the comparative one and is therefore preferable for general clinical use. Moreover, the patients appear to differ considerably in their ability to use the VAS reliably. When assessing efficacy of treatment, attention should therefore be paid to several complementary indices of pain relief as well as to the individual's tendency to bias his estimates.

Harvey R F, Jellinek H M 1983 Patient profiles: utilization in functional performance assessment. Archives of Physical Medicine and Rehabilitation 64: 268–271.
A computerized XY graphic plotted profile has been developed as a method of displaying patient progress and goals using the Patient Evaluation Conference System (PECS) as the data source. Each profile is a bar graph of functional status and goal scores for specific contact-evaluation points. Contacts are represented by different colors so that one color is superimposed on the other. Individual functional items are plotted on the X-axis at the appropriate level of independent or dependent function, as indicated by the 0–7 scale which appears on the Y-axis. The profile is used in goal-oriented team conferences,

and provides a focus on particular problems of low status or discrepancies between status and goals. This visual aid can provide a display of rehabilitation progress useful to the patient, family, and staff.

Linton S J, Melin L 1982 The accuracy of remembering chronic pain. Pain 13: 281–285.
Twelve chronic pain patients were employed in an investigation of the accuracy of memory for chronic pain. Subjects first made pain ratings before entering a treatment program. At dismissal 3–11 weeks later, they were asked to remember how much pain they had had at baseline. Results show that patients remembered having significantly more pain, than they actually rated during the baseline period. Caution is therefore warranted when using post-hoc pain measures with chronic pain patients.

Melzack R 1975 The McGill Pain Questionnaire: major properties and scoring methods. Pain 1: 277–299.
The McGill Pain Questionnaire consists primarily of 3 major classes of word descriptors — sensory, affective and evaluative — that are used by patients to specify subjective pain experience. The questionnaire was designed to provide quantitative measures of clinical pain that can be treated statistically. This paper describes the procedures for administration of the questionnaire and the various measures that can be derived from it.

C. SCANDINAVIAN CONTRIBUTIONS—EVALUATION OF PAIN

Bunkan B 1982 Psychomotoric treatment. Proceedings IX. International Congress of Physical Therapy, Stockholm, pp 213–220.
This paper describes the theory, the examination, and the treatment named 'psychomotoric treatment', which is a Norwegian somatopsychic treatment method. In this treatment, the whole body is taken into consideration, and it is used for muscular tension due to different life stresses where the problems are manifested in aches, stiffness and pain in the musculo-skeletal system.

Ljunggren A E 1983 Descriptions of pain and other sensory modalities in patients with lumbago-sciatica and herniated intervertebral discs. Interview administration of an adapted McGill Pain Questionnaire. Pain 16: 265–276.
This paper aims at elucidating to what extent patients with lumbago-sciatica in the presence of herniated intervertebral disc are inclined to describe their pain in a characteristic way. The description of herniation pain was represented by a variety of pain qualities. The mapping of pain seems to represent a diagnostic aid.

Roxendal G 1982 Clinical evaluation of body awareness training for patients with schizophrenia. Proceedings IX. International Congress of Physical Therapy, Stockholm, 227–231.
The paper describes the content and use of a Body Awareness Scale consisting of two parts: one concerning reported subjective information based on a structured interview and one concerning conservation of the patient's behaviour during the interview and the result of a structured movement test. A factor analysis of collected data and the results of a reliability test are reported.

Sundsvold M 1975 Muscular tension and psychopathology. Psychotherapy and Psychosomatics 26: 219–228.
The paper describes the results of the use of an earlier version of the GPM-method used in a study of four groups: a psychotic inpatient group, a neurotic inpatient group, a patient group from a physical therapy institute and a healthy

control group. Several differences were found between the groups which are helpful in treatment planning.

Sundsvold M, Vaglum P, Østberg B 1981 Movements, lumbar and temporomandibular pains and psychopathology. Psychotherapy and psychosomatics 35: 1–8.
The paper reports the results from the evaluation of passive and active movements in five body regions in both males and females in four psychodiagnostic groups. The psychotic group was most inhibited, followed by the ego-weak neurotic group, the substance abusing group and the healthy control group. Men were more inhibited than women in three regions, mostly in the lumbosacral region. Women were more significantly inhibited in the temporomandibular region.

Sundsvold M, Vaglum, P 1982 Muscle characteristics and psychopathology: I. A description of a reliable Global Physiotherapeutic Muscle examination method (GPM). Proceedings IX. International Congress of Physical Therapy, Stockholm.
The paper gives a short description of the background and composition of the GPM-examination method.

Sundsvold M, Vaglum P 1982 Muscle characteristics and psychopathology: II. Three studies of psychotic, ego-weak neurotic and drug abusing patients using the GPM-examination. Proceedings IX. International Congress of Physical Therapy, Stockholm.
The paper summarizes methods, materials and results from three different studies of groups with a different degree of psychopathology using the GPM-examination. The studies show that the GPM-examination method may discriminate between psychiatric patients with a different degree, type and course of psychopathology.

PART 2.
BEHAVIORAL AND PSYCHOLOGICAL APPROACHES TO PAIN

Fordyce W E 1976 Behavioural Methods for chronic pain and illness C.V. Mosby, St Louis.
An updated comprehensive review of pain as a learned behaviour and strategies for its treatment; this is the classic description of the behaviouralist approach to dealing with chronic pain.

Kosterlitz H W, Terenius L Y (eds) 1980 Pain and society (Dahlem Konferenzen, Nov 26–30, 1979) Verloy Chemic Weinhom.
A comprehensive review of experimental, clinical, ethical and philosophical aspects of pain is presented in this book.

Kramlinger K G, Swanson D W, Maruta T 1983 Are patients with chronic pain depressed? American Journal of Psychiatry 140: 747–749.
Of 100 consecutive patients treated in a program for management of chronic pain, 25 were definitely depressed, 39 were probably depressed, and 36 were not depressed. Comparisons between the definitely depressed and nondepressed groups showed them to have strikingly similar characteristics as well as treatment outcome. Nearly 90% of the definitely depressed patients showed resolution of their depression without use of antidepressant medication.

Marshall K 1981 'Pain relief in labour'. Physiotherapy 67(1): 8–11.
The role of the obstetric physiotherapist as part of a team helping prepare the

pregnant woman both physically and mentally for childbirth is described. Instruction and training is delivered in group sessions by the physiotherapist and midwife together. The interplay of pain and psychological stress is discussed and a method of psychoprophylaxis which alters established behaviour patterns and thereby aims to substitute new conditioned reflexes and 'raise the pain threshold' is outlined. As acknowledged in the article this method is based upon Pavlovian classical conditioning. Methods of physical preparation for labour are reviewed, consisting of active relaxation, controlled, conscious breathing, good postural disposition and neuromuscular techniques and skills. The 'pain relief' of the title is one of a number of positive results gained from the training described. As the author states, 'The aims of preparation for childbirth are to replace fear with understanding, negative responses with positive responses, chaos with discipline, and a passive role with an active role'.

Moon M H (in press 1984) The philosophy of pain. New Zealand Journal of Physiotherapy.
Western medicine is based on Cartesian dualism that effectively separated the mind from the body in a manner that allowed investigation of the anatomy of the body-machine without challenging theology. This concept no longer holds and the physiotherapist dealing with pain must use an integrated approach to treat the whole person within his social environment.

Pilowsky I 1976 The psychiatrist and the pain clinic. American Journal of Psychiatry 133:7.
A psychiatrist practicing in Adelaide, Australia, discusses the role of a psychiatrist in a pain clinic in introducing a multidimensional approach which is difficult for non-psychiatric clinicians to accept.

Pilowsky I, Spence N D 1983 Manual for the illness behaviour questionnaire (2nd edn) University of Adelaide, Australia.
This manual contains references leading to development of tests to identify those patients with chronic pain who are showing illness behaviour.

Shealy C N 1976 The pain game. Celestial Arts.
This is a useful book for patients and clinicians who want to view pain from other perspectives. The accent of treatment is on relaxation, physical fitness and education about pain.

Sternbach R A (ed) 1978 The psychology of pain. Raven Press, New York, 271pp.
A series of articles by twelve psychologists and behavioural scientists who have contributed to the psychological aspect of pain are presented here by one of the most well-known American pain psychologists. Topics include neurological, behavioural, perceptual, cognitive and clinical research studies.

PART 3.
TREATMENT APPROACHES: TENS, ACUPUNCTURE, MANUAL THERAPY, EMG BIOFEEDBACK
TENS

Frampton V M 1982 Pain control, with the aid of transcutaneous nerve stimulation. Physiotherapy 68(3): 77–81.
This paper discusses the use of TENS to relieve pain in peripheral nerve injuries. It emphasizes that success depends entirely on very careful technique and follow-up and a comprehensive rehabilitation programme including an adequate length of treatment. Avulsion lesions of the brachial plexus and

causalgia are discussed. Three disorders in the painful peripheral nerve condition are identified: on-going peripheral nerve discharges, abnormal central effects, and abnormal responses to sympathetic nervous drive. How each is tackled is discussed. Practical points regarding the application of TENS and precautions are covered. The other sections of the paper deal with the history and assessment of pain, quantitive analysis of pain, intensity of treatment and occupational therapy. Three case histories and the treatment in each case are described as well as a brief report of a study of seventy patients with severe peripheral nerve pain.

Gersh M R, Wolf S L, Rao V R 1980 Evaluation of transcutaneous electrical nerve stimulation for pain relief in peripheral neuropathy. Physical Therapy 60(1): 48–52.
A single case study is reported in which a patient with constant burning pain of both feet, with a history of heart disease and mild psychiatric disturbances, was evaluated and treated with TENS. Evaluation involved use of the McGill Pain Questionnaire, and treatment parameters are carefully described. The case study demonstrates the need for developing objective evaluation criteria and careful, rational protocols for TENS application.

Herman E 1977 The use of transcutaneous nerve stimulation in the management of chronic pain. Physiotherapy Canada 29: 65–71.
Transcutaneous nerve stimulation (TCS) as it concerns physiotherapists, is discussed. An outline of the role of pain clinics and the possible place of TCS in pain management are presented along with methods of application, necessary precautions and results of TCS trials on 207 chronic pain patients.

Mannheimer J S, Lampe G N 1984 Clinical transcutaneous electrical nerve stimulation. F.A. Davis, Philadelphia.
This book is the most comprehensive treatise on the subject of TENS and its role in pain management. It contains all the necessary information for the successful use of TENS by the clinician. The book includes chapters on the neurophysiology of pain, patient evaluation and post-operative applications. Numerous case studies, illustrations, literature review and references are presented.

Paxton S L 1980 Clinical uses of TENS. A survey of physical therapists. Physical therapy 60(1): 38–44.
The results of a survey of physical therapists in the U.S.A. who use TENS for treatment of various pain conditions revealed that about 65% of 196 respondents used TENS primarily for chronic rather than acute pain, and that short-term use of TENS was more effective than long-term use. A variety of other modalities were reported as used in conjunction with TENS, especially heat, exercise, and massage. How pain is usually evaluated was also reported with the most frequent means used and the patient's subjective estimation of relief.

Richardson R R, Meyer P R, Raimonde A J 1979 Transabdominal neuro-stimulation in acute spinal cord injuries. Spine 4: 47.
This paper discusses the role and use of TENS in patients with acute spinal cord injuries who were treated within 40 hours post onset and had no neurologic recovery below the lesion. Transabdominal TENS prevented the development of ileus, gastrointestinal hemorrhage or obstruction.

Smith C R, Lewith G T, Machin D 1983 Transcutaneous nerve stimulation and osteo-arthritic pain. Physiotherapy 69(8): 266–268.
The article reports a preliminary study to establish a controlled method of assessing transcutaneous nerve stimulation (TNS) as a treatment for the pain caused by osteo-arthritis (OA) of the knee. The authors state that the results of

the study substantially support the suggestion that brief intense stimulation
with TNS is a useful method of relieving pain in OA of the knee over a four-
week period. The study was single-blind, randomised, and each patient
received eight treatments over a four week period using either TNS or placebo
(a defunctioned TNS machine). At the end of the eight treatments, ten patients
(66.7%) in the TNS group and four patients (26.7%) in the placebo group
showed a significant pain relief ($\chi = 3.35$, df $= 1$, $p = 0.067$). A subjective
linear seven-point scale for pain assessment was used. Analgesic intake was
recorded daily as was sleep disturbance due to pain. 'Significant' pain relief is
defined.

Solomon R A, Viernstein M C, Long D M 1980 Reduction of postoperative pain
and narcotic use by transcutaneous electrical nerve stimulation. Surgery
87: 142.
The authors compared the effectiveness of TENS in the control of post-
operative pain specifically in the drug-naive and drug-experienced patient.
Benefit was most apparent in patients who were drug-naive.

Stratton S A, Smith M M 1980 Postoperative thoracotomy. Effect of
transcutaneous electrical nerve stimulation on forced vital capacity. Physical
Therapy 60(1): 45–47.
This study was aimed at determining if TENS aids post-op patients to breathe
more deeply after thoracic surgery. In 11 experimental subjects, forced vital
capacity did show improvement during the 10 minute interval of TENS
application, but that there was no carry over after TENS was discontinued. Ten
control subjects did not show any improved breathing capacity. Pain relief was
not measured.

Wolf S L, Gersh M, Rao V R 1981 Examination of electrode placements and
stimulation parameters in treating chronic pain with conventional
transcutaneous electrical nerve stimulation (T.E.N.S.). Pain 11:37.
An analysis of the results of TENS used with many patients is presented. The
paper highlights the need to use TENS early in the acute stage, stating that its
effectiveness decreases with the number of interventions that precede its use. It
discusses electrode placement techniques and the need to evaluate different
methods. Very few patients obtained optimal results with TENS at the time of
the initial application.

Acupuncture

Mann F 1977 Scientific aspects of acupuncture. William Heinemann, London.
This is one of at least six books written by a doctor with many years of
acupuncture experience in the West. The author describes it as an attempt to
explain certain aspects of acupuncture in terms of science.
It is interesting and contains may references to experimentation.

Multi Author 1979 Advances in acupuncture and acupuncture anaesthesia. The
Peoples Medical Publishing House, Beijing, China.
This is a compilation of abstracts of papers presented on the National
Symposium of Acupuncture, Moxibustion and Acupuncture Anaesthesia, held
in Beijing June 1–5, 1979. Its interest lies in the wide spectrum of diseases for
which acupuncture has been used.

History/geography of acupuncture

Duffin D H 1978 Acupuncture past and present. Physiotherapy 64(7): 203–07.
This is an account of acupuncture as practised in various countries of the world

including Great Britain, America, Canada, Europe, Russia, Korea and China. It mentions the earliest recordings of acupuncture treatments in some Western countries as well as current practices in China.

Evidence of effect of acupuncture

Lin M-T, Chandra A, Chen-Yen S-M, Chern Y-F 1980 Needle stimulation of acupuncture loci chu-chih (L1-II) and ho-ku (L1-4) induces hypothermia effects and analgesia in normal adults. American Journal of Chinese Medicine 9(1): 74–83.
This study on 18 healthy medical students, used acupuncture with intermittent manual 'twirling' at points on the colon meridian. The subjects were kept resting at fixed ambient temperature for one and a half to two hours prior to commencement of acupuncture. Needles were then inserted for 20 minutes after Teh Ch'i was noted and were 'twirled' every 5 minutes. Measurements were recorded at one minute intervals. Analgesia was measured by response to hot plate. Results showed: (a) a fall in oral temperature of average 0.6°C, (b) a fall in metabolic rate of average 7.1 w/kg, (c) a rise in cutaneous temperature of the arm of average 1.1°C, (d) no change in respiratory evaporative heat loss, and (e) an analgesic effect especially following stimulation of colon 4.

Okazaki N 1980 Analgesic effects of electroacupuncture upon experimental periostal and cutaneous pains. Matsui 29(8) 784–792 (English Abstract).
In this study 39 healthy volunteers were divided into two groups, one receiving experimentally induced periostal pain, and the other cutaneous pain. They were further divided into three groups — one received no acupuncture, one received electroacupuncture to the same side of the body as the noxious stimulus, and the third group received electroacupuncture to the opposite side. The results showed: (a) analgesic effect in both electroacupuncture groups but this was greater for cutaneous than periostal pain; (b) analgesia was more obvious in the ipsilateral group than the contralateral group; (c) analgesia was more obvious with higher intensity stimulation than with lower intensity.

Explanation of effect of acupuncture

Melzack R 1978 Pain mechanisms: Recent research. Acupuncture & Electro-therapeutic Research International Journal 3: 109–112.
This article comments on pain measurement in animals and man and refers to the McGill Pain Questionnaire as a reliable method in man. The author then describes the brain mechanisms which underlie pain and analgesia:
(a) somatotopic organization — different body areas are optimally analgesic at different levels of the dorsal-ventral plane. There are also optimal current intensities for each area to produce analgesia; (b) pharmacological basis — there are several neurochemical agents including serotonin and catecholamine systems which are active in analgesia. Transient and chronic pain may be perceived in different ways; (c) prolonged neural activity related to pain — the elicitation of after discharges following brain stimulation can produce analgesia outlasting the duration of the after discharges. Finally, Melzack mentions the gate control theory in relation to acupuncture and TENS and the correspondence between trigger points and acupuncture points.

Price P, Rees H 1982 The chemical basis of acupuncture analegesia. British Journal of Acupuncture 5(2): 13–15.
The authors supply evidence that opiate peptides are involved in acupuncture analgesia. They describe comparative studies on two groups of patients, one of whom suffered from chronic pain, the other from drug addiction. Both groups

were given electroacupuncture and the differences in the CSF levels of met-enkephalin and β endorphin following treatment are explained. Low frequency electroacupuncture may release β endorphin and high frequency releases met-enkephalin. Naloxone will block the former effect but not the latter. Serotonin seems to play a more important role in the effects of high frequency than low frequency electroacupuncture. The short-term chemical changes observed do not explain the long term relief of pain.

Methods used in acupuncture

Cho M-H, Cho C, 1977 A simple physiological method of isolating the topographical correspondence between somatic areas and auricular points, and the clinical application of this method for the pain treatment. Acupuncture & Electro-therapeutic Research International Journal 3: 113–120.
This describes a method of using a pulse generating electric stimulating machine to locate and treat the correspondence between a somatic area and ear point. A needle attached to the positive electrode of the machine is inserted into the centre of the area of pain. The negative electrode is attached to a smooth-tipped needle. With current turned on, the smooth-tipped needle is used to locate the point of correspondence by sliding on the ear surface. When a sensation of pulsation occurs either at the ear or the area of pain, the correct correspondence has been found. The sliding needle should be kept at this point for approximately 7 seconds by which time most of the pain should have gone. The auricular points are rarely bigger than 0.1 mm.

Treatment—acupuncture

Cardiovascular Section, Acupuncture Research Institute, Academy of Traditional, Chinese Medicine. 1981 Acupuncture in coronary heart disease. Chinese Medical Journal 94 (2): 81–84.
This describes 44 cases treated with several courses of acupuncture therapy, each course lasting 10 days. Marked improvement was noted in 65.9% and occurred after 10 days. Improvement was noted in 29.5%. The symptoms which improved were precordial pain, cardiac hypofunction, shortness of breath, palpitation. ECG after between 1–3 months' treatment showed marked improvement in 20% of affected patients and improvement in 43.6%.

Gunn C C 1976 Transcutaneous neural stimulation, needle acupuncture & 'Teh Ch'i' phenomenon. American Journal of Acupuncture 4 (4): 317–321.
Teh Ch'i, or needle sensation, occurs within seconds following needle acupuncture when mechanical or electrical stimulation is applied. Successful therapy results when Teh Ch'i is experienced. In TENS treatment for low back pain, best results are obtained when the electrodes are placed over motor points or major nerve trunks. If the gate control theory remains valid, the contribution of large diameter afferent fiber activity from the deep muscle nerve supply is more significant than that from superficial cutaneous nerves. The efficacy of Ho-Ku point (first dorsal interosseous) is probably related to its high afferent innervation ratio. Teh Ch'i does not occur in cutaneous stimulation. It occurs best when a needle is inserted and stimulated at the muscle zone of innervation or when TNS produces visible muscle contraction.

Gunn C C, Milbrandt W E 1977 Tennis elbow and acupuncture. American Journal of Acupuncture 5 (1): 61–66.
The authors point out that accurate diagnosis of these cases is essential as those that prove resistant to treatment are often those with referred symptoms from a

cervical spine lesion. These cases are classified as Type V tennis elbow. Acupuncture treatment in types I-IV (Cyriax) tennis elbow consists of needle insertion to tender points in the elbow region. It is important to achieve Teh Ch'i. Best results are obtained when all points belonging to both anterior and posterior rami are treated. In Type V tennis elbow, acupuncture to points around the neck, shoulder, arm, medial epicondyle and hand is often necessary. Relief of symptoms should occur 4–5 weeks after the nerve roots are free, although if Wallerian degeneration has occurred at least 12 weeks are necessary.

Kisoshita 1979 Mechanism and application of paraneural acupuncture for neuralgia. British Journal of Acupuncture 2 (1):37.
This study was conducted in Tokyo, Japan. The author notes three effects of acupuncture during treatment for painful conditions: (a) increase in skin and muscle temperature by 1° C in the effected side of the body. Prior to treatment this side was noted to be 1° C lower in temperature than the normal side; (b) increase of over 50% in pulse wave amplitude in the limb receiving acupuncture; (c) alleviation of muscle contracture. The author contends that neuralgia pain may often be relieved by relaxing the muscles which surround the nerve path supplying the muscles. Acupuncture to the points around the nerve radix or motor point will achieve this. His results with paraneural acupuncture for trigeminal neuralgia, sciatica, lumbago, cervico-brachial syndrome and intercostal neuralgia are all very good.

Lu G W 1983 Neurobiologic research on acupuncture in China as exemplified by acupuncture analgesia. Anaesthesia and Analgesia 62: 235–240.
The research being done in China is concentrated on acupuncture analgesia. The results of studies fall into 3 categories: (a) Nervous system mechanisms: studies have shown more pressure and stretch receptors in the area of acupuncture points than non-acupuncture points. Studies in different parts of China and in Japan have shown contrasting results in the type of nerve fiber responsible for acupuncture signal transmission. Researchers in Jilin have shown that electroacupuncture will inhibit pain sensitive cells in the spinal trigeminal nucleus. Many studies have demonstrated the part played by the raphe nucleus or medial reticular formation, and caudate and thalamic nuclei in acupuncture analgesia. (b) Neurohumoral factors: serotonin and endogenous opiates are important in analgesia. Both inorganic chemicals and amino acids are thought to play an important role. (c) Meridian lines: in people sensitive to acupuncture, stimulatation of one point can cause erythema or ordema in many other points on the same meridian. Some researchers dispute the possibility of a meridian system separate to the known nervous system.

Lu G, Xie J, Yang, J, Wang Y, Wang Q 1981. Afferent nerve fiber composition at point Zusanli in relation to acupuncture analgesia. Chinese Medical Journal 94 (4): 255–263.
This article describes the methods and results of examining and comparing Zusanli (Stomach 36 which is inferior to the anterior aspect of the knee), Quchi (colon 11 which is at the elbow) and a non-meridian point (0.5 cm lateral to Zusanli) in animals. Results showed the following: (a) marked analgesia was obtained only when the pain source was situated at the same segment of innervation as point Zusanli; (b) the difference in analgesic effect between point Zusanli and the two other points was statistically very significant; (c) the main large fibers, especally $A\beta\gamma$, are activated when highly effective analgesic foci are stimulated which is not the case when control foci are stimulated; (d) at Zusanli there were 22% Group I fibers, 52% Group II, and 26% Group III fibers; (e) the mean values of the ratio of myelinated to non-myelinated fibers in meridian points as opposed to the non-meridian point showed a statistically significant difference.

Takeshige C 1980 Individual effectiveness of acupuncture analgesia and endogenous morphine-line factors. British Journal of Acupuncture 3 (2):38.
This describes studies in Tokyo, Japan. The effectiveness of acupuncture analgesia was examined in rats, and shown to be present in approximately 50% of these animals. The rats were then grouped into acupuncture effective and non-effective categories. The amount of endogenous morphine-like factors in the whole brain except cerebellum was 25 times greater in the acupuncture effective group than in the non-effective group. Periaqueduct central gray stimulation induced analgesia was also obvious only in the acupuncture effective group. Morphine was also much more effective in the acupuncture effective group. Intraperitoneal injection of 250 mg/kg of d-phenylalanine, an inhibitor of morphine-like factors polypeptidase, reversed the acupuncture non-effective group to acupuncture effective.

Zhang A, Pan X, Xu S, Cheng J, Mo W 1980 Endorphins and acupuncture analgesia. Chinese Medical Journal 93 (10): 673–680.
Electroacupuncture significantly increases human CSF endorphins fraction 1, III and 29. Post-acupuncture release of endorphins was observed in the periaqueductal gray, caudate nucleus and accumbens nucleus.
Electroacupuncture increases the pain threshold in rabbits, and inhibits the cortical potentials evoked by tooth pulp stimulation in rabbits. Naloxone will reverse the effect of moderate strength electroacupuncture, but not of super strength electroacupuncture, suggesting that the methods of analgesia differ.

Manual therapy

Brodin H 1979 Principles of examination and treatment in manual medicine. Scandinavian Journal of Rehabilitation Medicine 11: 181–187.
General principles for testing of pain and mobility are discussed. Different active and passive mobilization procedures are described, and examples are given of when each of them is most appropriate.

Brodin H 1982 Inhibition-facilitation technique for lumbar pain treatment. Manuelle Medizine 20: 95–98.
Out of 41 patients examined with manual therapy techniques, 21 patients were found to have more then one painful and rigid lumbar segment. These patients were treated mainly with an active facilitation-inhibition technique below the limit of pain. A correlation between a reduction of pain and increase of mobility was demonstrated in this study.

Coxhead C E, Inskip H, Meade T W, North W R S, Troup J D G 1981 Multicentre trial of physiotherapy in the management of sciatic symptoms. The Lancet 1: 8229. 1065–1068.
This is an account of a randomised controlled study that looked at a number of treatments used either singly or in combination. Patients with pain of sciatic distribution with or without neurological deficit were randomly allocated to traction, manipulation, exercises, corset or a control treatment consisting of shortwave diathermy and a back lecture. There was some benefit from manipulation but, more importantly, there was a statistically significant increase in symptomatic improvement with an increasing number of treatments used in combination. This was complemented by a clear tendency for those patients who received fewer types of treatments during the trial to have further treatment during the ensuing three months. None of the clinical characteristics of the patients in this study was associated with a tendency to do well or badly with a particular treatment.

Cyriax J H 1982 Textbook of orthopaedic medicine, Vol I. Bailliere Tindall, London.
This book presents orthopaedic medicine, which would be better referred to as orthopaedic dysfunction. Cyriax's differential evaluation of extremity pain, particularly by the methods of selective tension, are invaluable clinically. His writing is clear and quite concise. Of all the texts on orthopaedic examination, this is the most helpful to clinical physical therapists. In the spinal section of this book, he appears to abandon his well thought-out system of 'differential diagnosis' and resorts instead to describing nearly all back pain as coming from the intervertebral disc.

Gonnella C, Paris S V, Kutner M 1982 Reliability in evaluating passive intervertebral motion. Physical Therapy 62 (4): 436–444.
In this article the authors evaluate the subjective sensation of palpating passive intervertebral joint motion. The motion was scaled on a 7-point system from 0 to 6. The findings were that experienced and trained manual therapists had a high level of consistency when grading the same joint on the same patient at separate visits. Where the reliability was less than satisfactory, the different examiners examining the same joint tended to grade it somewhat differently. As a result, one can conclude that until a better training model is available, passive intervertebral motion testing is reliable only for the clinician wishing to detect either an increase or decrease in the range of motion following treatment.

Grieve G P 1982 Neck traction. Physiotherapy 68: 8. 260–265.
The use of cervical traction is presented, following the general principle that traction is simply another way of using movement to treat painful abnormalities of movement. Provided its use is controlled, carefully assessed and precisely recorded it forms a valuable and effective treatment. Included for discussion are the effects of traction, measurement, recording and precautions. One of the principle themes explored is that of the mechanism whereby traction achieves its effect upon pain and restricted movement. The argument presented is that it is not solely by way of vertebral separation but by a complex of different effects, and both experimental evidence and clinical experience are used in the discussion. This greater field of physiological and anatomical effects opens a much wider application of this useful treatment method.

Grieve G P 1983 The hip. Physiotherapy 69: 6 196–204.
The article discusses the management of patients with painful and functionally disturbed hip joints whose condition falls short of warranting hip replacement. Prior to discussing examination, techniques of treatment and re-education, the author presents a condensed discussion of the joint under the headings: epidemiology, comparative anatomy, biomechanics, vascularity, aetiology and clinical features. A well-argued case is made, and supported by a wide selection of relevant reference material, (a) that currently minor degrees of arthrosis discovered early by meticulous examination techniques can and should be treated sooner, probably with better long-term results and (b) that treatment should include passive mobilising techniques to relieve pain, free restricted movement and improve function in the early painful hip. While other modalities of treatment are noted in passing, it is the use of passive movement procedures backed up by careful muscle re-education and home exercises which form the main part of the second half of the article.

Hoppenfeld 1976 Physical examination of the spine and extremities. Appleton-Century Crofts, New York.
This is an excellent book, not so much for joint examination, as the title suggests, but for surface anatomy and palpation. Whereas Cyriax makes little reference to palpation, pointing out that it can be extremely misleading, Hoppenfeld deals almost entirely with palpation, neglecting most other aspects

of evaluation. This is a book on palpation and thanks to the fine artwork of Hugh Thomas, it is the best on the topic.

Ljunggren A E et al 1984 Autotraction versus manual traction in patients with prolapsed lumbar intervertebral discs. Scandinavian Journal of Rehabilitation Medicine (in press).
A study is reported where 49 patients with comparable anamnestic and clinical data were randomized for autotraction and manual traction. The two types of traction are discussed, and are found to be equally efficient. If traction is given for hospital patients manual traction is preferred. Pain was reduced, and one quarter of the patients avoided surgery. The symptoms did not return within a two-year period.

Maitland G D 1980 Peripheral manipulation. Butterworth, London.

Maitland G D 1968 Vertebral manipulation. Butterworth, London.
These two texts represent a milestone in the development of manual therapy methods. Maitland took a little-known technique of oscillation, defined four grades of it and went on to collect the clinical experience so well expressed in his writings. Oscillations are an excellent method for treating joint pain and have been shown to work most effectively in the early stages of a painful joint disorder. However, he applies these to the actual range of motion without particular thought to the end-feels or to the accessory movements of the joint.

Maitland G D 1983 Treatment of the glenohumeral joint by passive movement. Physiotherapy. 69: 1. 3–7.
The article describes how any patient referred for physiotherapy whose pain can be reproduced by passive movement can be treated by the methods described. The methods consist of passive accessory and physiological movements, used either in a painfree part of the available joint range into the beginning of the painful range or at the limit of a physiological range. Patients are grouped according to their signs and symptoms rather than by diagnoses related to pathology. The four main groups include patients unable to move the shoulder because of pain, those restricted by pain and stiffness, those in which pain is momentary and sharp and those in which limitation of movement is related to stiffness rather than pain. Only the principles of treatment are discussed and reference is made to the author's textbooks on the subject.

Moritz U 1979 Evaluation of manipulation and other manual therapy. Scandinavian Journal of Rehabilitation Medicine 11: 173–179.
This article is a review of the literature dealing with the effect of manual therapy treatment on the spine and the extremities. The most prominent symptoms for the greater number of patients are pain upon movement and weight-bearing. Difficulties in obtaining valid results of treatment are stressed. Mobility, muscle strength—and in non-painful conditions—and functional capacity related to social life and work, are used as criteria for improvement. The review states that manipulation of the lumbar spine might have an immediate short-term effect on low back pain in a limited number of patients, but has no superior long-term effect as compared to other methods of treatment. However, further research is needed, especially case reports where more information is given regarding the specific manipulation technique that is used relative to the patient's clinical signs. It is also important that the treatment technique is carried out by well-trained and experienced persons. Manual therapy in decreased mobility of the extremity joints has received support from a few controlled studies. The risk for injury to joints in inflammatory, destructive joint disease appears to be less than in conventional mobilization.

O'Donoghue C E 1984 'Treatment of back pain'. Physiotherapy 70: 1. 7–8.
This article briefly reviews some of the recent research published on the

treatment of low back pain. It makes the point that since a number of the investigations published in recent years are based on work done by physiotherapists and relate to aspects of clinical management this should be reflected in current practice. The results of the research considered in this paper are briefly summarised under the headings: start of therapy, different therapies, number of treatments and education. The conclusions it draws under these headings are: (a) that physiotherapists should be free to select the treatment of their choice for the patient; (b) that there is a suggestion that more than one treatment has a beneficial effect and there is mounting evidence that manipulation should be one modality to be included; (c) that there should be an adequate amount of education included as part of therapy; (d) that patients respond better when therapy is instituted early rather than late; (e) that maximum benefit occurs during the first month of treatment.

Rasmussen G G 1979 Manipulation in treatment of low back pain (a randomized clinical trial). Manuelle Medizine 1: 8–10.
This controlled trial is performed in a clinically well defined group of patients. The group had 24 male patients between 20–50 years with a mean age of 34.9 years, with low back pain for less than 3 weeks without any sign of root pressure. They were treated with either short wave or manipulation 3 times a week for 14 days. The patients were declared fully restored if they had no pain, normal function, no objective signs of disease and were fit to work. Contrary to what is reported by several authors, Rasmussen found that 92% of the patients treated with manipulation improved, whereas only half of the patients receiving short wave improved. All restored patients were free of symptoms for at least one year.

Steindler A 1977 Kinesiology of the human body under normal and pathological conditions, Thomas, Springfield, Illinois.
Before a joint can be adequately examined, the function, both normal and pathological but particularly normal function, must be clearly understood. Steindler has meticulously examined the motion of extremity joints, spine and rib cage. With this knowledge, it is much easier to decide not only where but what is limiting motion in a joint. As a result, the clincian no longer tries to, for instance, straighten an elbow by pulling on the forearm, but recognizes that the capability of elbow action includes adduction, radius sliding down on ulna, and radius and ulna rolling inwards on one another. It is these components that should be mobilized, and when successfully completed, elbow extension should be free.

EMG Biofeedback and treatment for painful spasticity

Finch L, Harvey J 1983 Factors associated with shoulder-hand syndrome in hemiplegia: clinical survey. Physiotherapy Canada 35: 145–148.
Unknown predisposing factors resulting in the development of shoulder-hand-syndrome in hemiplegic patients, led investigators to conduct a four-month survey of recent stroke patients in an acute-care hospital. A dependency on others for aid, diminished sensory awareness, poor shoulder joint integrity and a diminished mental status were the major characteristics of hemiplegics with this shoulder problem. The need for the development of better functional aid and shoulder support is clearly evident from this survey.

Gowland C 1982 Recovery of motor function following stroke: profile and predictors. Physiotherapy Canada 34: 77–84.
Two hundred and twenty-nine stroke patients admitted to a rehabilitation centre were studied in order to develop predictors of performance outcomes for

stroke patients undergoing rehabilitation. Four aspects of physical recovery of the arm and leg, the gait and level of gross motor performance were measured. Predictions regarding the outcome of the hemiplegic leg, gait and gross motor performance were found to be of use. None of the characteristics investigated, however, were found to be useful predictors of the performance outcome of the hemiplegic arm.

Jones A L, Wolf S L 1980 Treating low back pain. EMG biofeedback training during movement. Physical Therapy 60(1): 58–63.
A single case study is reported of a patient with chronic low back pain of two year's duration. EMG biofeedback training for muscle relaxation was used after a thorough evaluation. EMG activity in the painful muscle groups during specific movements were analyzed as a means of evaluating the effectiveness of the treatment. After 15 sessions of biofeedback training over a five-week period, impressive pain relief was noted on pain ratings.

Peat M, Grahame R E 1977 Shoulder function in hemiplegia. A method of electromyographic and electrogoniometric analysis. Physiotherapy Canada 29: 131–137
The electrical activity of the shoulder muscles was evaluated during raising and lowering of the arm in 30 normal subjects and 21 subjects with hemiplegia. The analysis of the two groups produced information of value in determining appropriate treatment procedures. In addition, the authors recommend frequent re-assessment of these muscles, in order to evaluate the effect and appropriateness of various therapeutic modalities used for pain reduction and increasing range of movement.

Savage R, Robertson L 1982 The relationship between adult hemiplegic shoulder, pain and depression. Physiotherapy Canada 34: 86–90.
The lack of knowledge regarding the etiology of adult hemiplegic shoulder pain is discussed and the question raised as to its relationship to the psychological factor of depression. A study was designed and depression, as assessed by physiotherapists, was found to have a statistically significant relationship with pain.

Stangel L 1975 The value of cryotherapy and thermotherapy in the relief of pain. Physiotherapy Canada 27: 135–139.
An extensive review of the literature on the physiological effects of heat and cold, as utilized clinically, is presented. These effects are considered in terms of pain relief and the mechanisms by which this is achieved. It is recommended that therapists should be involved in clinical research to prove or disprove the validity of modalities used for reduction of pain.

PART FOUR
COMPREHENSIVE TREATMENT OF CHRONIC PAIN

Andersson G 1979 Low back pain in industry: epidemiological aspects. Scandinavian Journal of Rehabilitation Medicine 11: 163–168.
The purpose of this survey was to summerize studies on frequency of low back pain in Sweden and to make conclusions and analyze relationships between back symptoms, work factors and individual factors.

Bergquist-Ullman M, Larsson U 1977 Acute low back pain in industry. Acta Orthopaedica Scandinavica, Supplement 170.
In this prospective study over three years the back school was found superior to a variety of manipulative procedures with regard to absence from work. With regard to the patients experience of pain, the back school was found

equal to physiotherapy, but both these groups were significantly better in this respect than the third group that received weak short wave diathermy.

Biering-Sörensen Fin 1983 A prospective study of low back pain in a general population: 1 Occurrence, recurrence and aetiology. Scandinavian Journal of Rehabilitation Medicine 15: 71–79.
928 men and women aged.30–60 underwent a lower back examination and were followed up after 12 months. Life-time prevalence for LBP for men was 65–70% and rose with increasing age from 62% to 81% among women. Heavy lifting, twisting and trauma were the most commonly stated causes.

Biering-Sörensen Fin 1983 A prospective study of low back pain in a general population: 2 Location, character, aggravating and relieving factors. Scandinavian Journal of Rehabilitation Medicine 15: 81–88.
This paper focus primarily on the 62% of the participants who reported previous and present LBP. The location and character of the pain is described. The aggravating factor was stooping followed by the sitting position.

Cairns D, Thomas L, Pace J B 1976 Comprehensive treatment approach to chronic low back pain. Pain 2: 301–308.
A comprehensive treatment program for chronic disability related to back disease is presented. This program used not only more traditional methods of medical care for the structural disabilities of chronic mechanical back disorders, but also used principles of active patient participation in the improvement process. The patients are educated in the manifestations of pain behavior and in the phase II treatment program emphasis on pain sources is downgraded to allow positive reinforcement for healthy behavior to develop. By use of an organized team approach, a significant number of patients can be processed; and an overall reduction in use of alternative medical resources has occurred.

Chapmen S L, Brena S F, Bradfore L A 1981 Treatment outcome in a chronic pain rehabilitation program. Pain 11: 255–268.
One hundred patients were selected who had completed an outpatient rehabilitation program designed to teach competent coping with chronic pain. Data at follow-up periods averaging 21 months post-treatment indicated statistically significant decreases in subjective pain intensity and increases in activities of daily living with substantial reductions in use of medications for pain. Changes from pretreatment to follow-up were not significantly different amoung groups of patients with pending, current, or no disability. Eight of 19 unemployed persons who had pending disability claims had returned to work at follow-up. It was concluded that considerable changes in function can occur with relatively brief outpatient pain rehabilitation and that pending or current disability is not necessarily an indication of likely treatment failure.

Hallett E C, Pilowsky I 1982 The response to treatment in a multidisciplinary pain clinic. Pain 12: 365–374.
Reports of the results obtained by multidisciplinary pain clinics are reviewed. The outcome of management of a cohort of patients referred to the Royal Adelaids Hospital Pain Clinic described. 37% of patients reported partial or complete relief. The problems of assessing outcome are discussed, as well as the difficulty of making meaningful comparisons between pain clinics. The evidence thus far available suggests that multidisciplinary pain clinics make a useful and important contribution to the management of pain syndromes.

Hayne C R 1984 Ergonomics and back pain. Physiotherapy 70: 1. 9–13.
This article reviews some aspects of ergonomics related to back pain in the light of the experience of the author. Manual handling and lifting, work postures and spinal supports are the headings used to summarise and discuss some of the more important investigations which have been undertaken. A few

investigations are considered in greater detail as examples of ergonomic studies
giving clinically relevant information for physiotherapists to utilize as part of
their total management of low back pain.

Lankhorst G 1983. The effect of the Swedish back school in chronic idiopathic
low back pain. Scandinavian Journal of Rehabilitation Medicine 15: 141–145.
In this prospective controlled study 43 patients were repeatedly tested for one
year. After one year no statistically significant positive effect of the back school
could be observed compared with the control group. Given the proven efficacy
of the back school in (sub)acute LBP, it should be administered when it is
most beneficial, i.e. in the early phase of LBP.

Malmgren S, Andersson G 1976 På jakt efter hälsoprofilen. (in swedish).
Socialmed inst. Universitet i Linköping.
Absence due to sickness for 1313 employees of Saab Scania, Linköping Sweden
in the age group 50–59 years is mainly a problem of long-term absence of a
minority of employees with an ever-increasing rate of absence. The single risk
factor that showed the strongest connection with absenteeism was a low degree
of physical activity during free time.

Myrnerts G 1982 The Saab Scania back-school: an evaluation. Proceedings from
the IX International Congress for Physical Therapy, Stockholm, Sweden
p 553–555.
The results of two evaluations of the Saab Scania back-school is presented and
analysed. The investigations showed that the back-school can improve exercise
habits, that practical training is more important than theoretical education and
that it is essential that the physical therapist follows up her back-school
students at their work places.

Nachemsson A 1979 A critical look at the treatment for low back pain.
Scandinavian Journal of Rehabilitation Medicine 11: 143–147.
To start early treatment seems to be a more important factor than the actual
modality itself. Futhermore, any type of attempted treatment should be
supplemented by a physical therapist teaching proper body mechanics and
ergonomics.

Oscarsson B 1982 The role of the occupational physiotherapist in swedish
company health service. Proceedings from the IX International Congress for
Physical Therapy, Stockholm, Sweden, p 550–552.
The Swedish company health service is described along with the different
preventive and curative duties of the physical therapist. Practical examples of
ergonomic work within industry are given.

Ready L B, Sarkis E, Turner J A 1982 Self-reported vs. actual use of medications
in chronic pain patients. Pain 12: 285–294.
Inappropriate or excessive medication use is a commonly observed problem
among patients with chronic pain. Comparing patients' self-reported drug use
with actual observed drug use, this study examines the incidence, nature and
magnitude of drug utilization in a selected population of pain patients and
evaluates the reliability of patient estimates of their own drug use. The data
support the clinical observation that patients with chronic pain tend to
underestimate their medication use. This tendency is greater for narcotic
analgesics than for a variety of other medications taken for pain and is greater
for women than men.

Roesch R, Ulrich D E 1980 Physical therapy management in the treatment of
chronic pain. Physical Therapy 60(1): 53–57.
This article describes a pain clinic program for treatment of chronic pain.
Major components are physical medicine and psychiatry. Components of the

physical therapy management are: evaluation, general body conditioning, self-regulation, patient education, and a home program. The approach is a behaviouralist one, emphasizing learning to live and function despite pain.

Turner J A, Calsyn D A, Fordyce W E, Ready L B 1982 Drug utilization patterns in chronic pain patients. Pain 12: 357–363.
In the population of chronic pain patients seen at multidisciplinary pain clinics excessive and/or inappropriate medication use is a frequent problem. This study examined differences between chronic pain patients who used no addicting medication (30% of the sample of 131 patients), those who used narcotic but not sedative medications (33%) and those who used both narcotic and sedative medications (37%). Narcotic-sedative using patients reported more physical impairment than the other two groups yet pain ratings for intensity did not differ, nor did sleeping/waking time. The no addicting drug group reported less spread of pain than the other two groups. Using the MMPI, the narcotic-sedative group scored highest on Lie, hypochondriasis, and hysteria scales.

Wickström G 1978. Effect of work on degenerative back disease. Scandinavian Journal of Work, Enviroment and Health 4 suppl 1, 1–12.
In this review the occupational back load factors were examined. Low back pain develops from a combination of hereditary and environmental causes. Specific factor such as injury, heavy lifting, stooped posture, and whole body vibration seem to contribute to the degenerative process. To prevent unnecessary pain and to avoid lost workdays efforts should be made to improve occupational health in the work place.

Index